*medicare
and the american rhetoric
of reconciliation*

medicare
and the american rhetoric
of reconciliation

BY
MAX J. SKIDMORE

UNIVERSITY OF ALABAMA PRESS
University, Alabama

For Joey

Among the many to whom gratitude is
due, I wish especially to thank my
son, Max Joseph Skidmore, Jr., for
his assistance in various capacities.

M. J. S.

contents

*medicare
and the american rhetoric of reconciliation
of reconciliation*

the american ideology

In the decade of the Great Depression of the 1930's, it became increasingly evident to more and more people that economic individualism and political liberties were not of themselves sufficient to ensure economic well-being for all in a complex society. This awareness, however, served more to permit American acceptance of increased governmental welfare activities than to change the traditional concepts of individual responsibility that had hindered the energetic solution of social problems from the beginnings of American industrialism. Writers frequently observe that the sway of an ideology no longer suited to the times has prevented, retarded, or distorted the development of many needed social welfare programs in the United States. Remarkably, those programs that have been established—social security is a major example—generally have found ready acceptance by the American people without greatly altering the main currents of an ideology that would seem to require their rejection.

This is not to say that the Great Depression did not lead to changes in outlook or in ideology. There were a number of significant changes, such as an increasing preoccupation with "security" and an increasing acceptance of overt governmental action to aid the economy ("priming the pump"). Nevertheless, as David Potter points out, we must be aware of the strands of continuity in our history as well as of the shifts and new departures. He notes that in spite of the historical emphasis upon laissez-faire, it was never the only guide to practical action; one of the key principles had always been the use of the government to make accessible to the public the economic abundance of the nation. The tactics changed during the depression; the principle did not.[1] Whether or not Potter's thesis of abundance is adequate, he is certainly correct in noting that one need not deny the existence of a major transformation in order to recognize a fundamental continuity.

An example of both change and continuity may be seen in the "Four Freedoms" declaration of President Franklin D. Roosevelt. "Freedom" has always been a cardinal tenet of the American ideology, and when the President proclaimed the "freedom of speech" and "freedom of religion" he was thoroughly in accord with American tradition. But when he went on to speak of "freedom from want" and "freedom from fear" he was, in a sense, departing from that tradition—or, rather, enlarging upon it. He added "two parts security under the label of 'freedom' " to the conception of freedom in the "classic liberal sense." [2] That is, he had embraced new ideas and practices but had, by rhetorical means, linked them with tradition.

In 1930 "Clinch Calkins" (Mrs. Charles Marquis Merrell of Philadelphia, a professional writer) indicted the traditional attitudes in a book ironically titled *Some Folks Won't Work*. There were several "widely held ideas about unemployment" which the book attempted to dispel. One was that unemployment comes only in hard times; another, that during unemployment the only sufferers are those who have been "too shiftless to save"; and a third, called by Calkins the most pervasive, "that if a man really wants to find work, he can find it . . ." [3] Though these attitudes had become obviously incompatible with reality, not even the Depression was adequate to change completely the orientation that they had produced over so long a time.

Reflecting the frontier heritage, the typical American had viewed with contempt the idea of government "doles" or "handouts." Influenced by a Puritan ethic that had stressed the sanctity of work, the typical American tended to believe that the acceptance of government funds indicated a personal flaw in the recipient that was detrimental to his morals, if not to his morale. Only the "large-scale financial or industrial buccaneer" could gain "something for nothing" without also gaining public scorn.[4] This was because he fulfilled the definition of the "true American" according to the traditional American ideology; he was an individualist, a materialist, a pragmatist, and—probably most important of all—he was a success.

During World War II, Karl Mannheim described the American culture in a way that showed divergent strains existing simultaneously. He pointed out that though the "Herbert Hoover type of rugged individualism" died with the Depression, the controls of the community remained loose, and the state and its functionaries remained in low esteem. He believed that American demands for freedom from all restrictions, and the traditional American attitude of being "agin the government" (some of which "is necessary in any successful Democracy") survived the depression with sufficient strength to engender social conflict. Nevertheless, the public accepted the New Deal efforts to embark upon programs using "democratic planning techniques," and training "a new type of administrative management personnel." [5] This is a good illustration of paradox in American culture, though neither especially new nor startling.

No investigation of American society can proceed very far without confronting the concept of the American character. As David Potter says, the existence of an American character is a major historical assumption. He chides historians, however, with failing to define the concept with "rigor and precision" —with failing to agree upon what they mean by the concept or upon what qualities should be considered as composing the national character. He observes a "striking evidence of the lack of adequate analysis." [6] He notes that the behavioral scientist has found that three of the most significant subjects for investigation are the "nursery, the bathroom, and the bedroom" and that the historian has been unable "to align his historical sights on these targets." [7]

Potter, too, assumes the existence of an American character. His argument, moreover, implies that it is susceptible to precise definition and that its definition would profit from an analysis of individual thought and from observation of individual behavior. This approach presupposes that "character" is an entity that can be observed, weighed, and measured, that it is composed of parts (persons) that are relatively interchangeable, and that it is no more than the sum of its parts. This approach seems to be an oversimplification, at best.

Henry Steele Commager, from the viewpoint of the historian, notes that Americans created a national character and formulated an American philosophy during a period of two and a half centuries. "That character," he writes, all but eludes description and that philosophy definition, yet both were unmistakable." [8] He shows that there is more to the historian's concept of the American character than a critic such as Potter has recognized, and that "the American character, as delineated by Tocqueville, Bryce, and Brogan at half-century intervals, seems substantially the same: the differences are quantitative and material rather than qualitative and moral." [9]

Reuel Denney has defined national character with somewhat more precision. His definition is perceptive, and probably is as specific as possible without introducing distortion through oversimplification. He says first that it does not refer to "constitutional personality types" or to their national distribution; second, that a " 'certain homogeneity' cannot be exhaustively explained by reference to non-characterological concepts of the society such as social structure, culture, and world view." [10] Though "learned behavior" may be too restrictive, this definition seems to be the best available. Keeping Denney's definition in mind when reading the historian's treatment of national character will tend to offset much of the uneasiness caused by Potter's criticism of the historical method.

All the scholars who have studied the period of the Great Depression and the New Deal point to the striking changes resulting within the American culture from the exigencies of internationalism and modern industrialism. Nevertheless, most of these scholars have also recognized the strains of continuity and the nature of the responses as elements in a developing pattern of American thought and experience. This is not to deny that a "revolution" of sorts took place, but to insist that the "revolutionary" changes themselves had roots deep in the society, and that much of the traditional survived unscathed.

Commager traces the development of the American character from the earliest times and makes it clear that paradox was not confined to the post-Depression years. In discussing the wide gap between 19th century political practice and 18th century constitutional patterns, he notes perceptively: "It was scarcely to be expected that a people as sentimental and as conservative as the Americans would give up their traditional principles or that a people as ingenious and adaptable as the Americans would abandon their necessary practices. They were neither to be frightened away from their symbols nor reasoned out of their habits." He observes that the people "very sensibly" chose both an official and an unofficial government, to be used for "ceremonial" or for "workaday" purposes, as appropriate.[11]

This reaction was duplicated during the Great Depression when the public, while retaining many of the tenets of the traditional American ideology, adopted programs that were clearly inconsistent with these tenets. The changes in outlook and ideology, though great, were not sufficiently so to require that the new practices be supported by a consistent and comprehensive ideological foundation. Certain ideological bases were advanced for each program, but many of these were merely rationalizations in terms of the traditional American ideology. From the late 19th century to the middle of the 20th, the material circumstances of the United States had greatly changed. "Yet it is by no means clear that this material change precipitated or even embraced a comparable change in the intellectual outlook or in the national character." [12]

From certain points of view, the New Deal was undeniably revolutionary; from others, it was not. From any viewpoint, its pragmatism and its general disregard of ideology were typical American responses to crisis situations. Franklin D. Roosevelt was first elected on a platform calling for a balanced budget. He "tirelessly reiterated" his aim of saving capitalism, and emphasized that most of his "revolutionary" changes were even milder than many similar programs in Great Britain that had long been approved by the British Tories.[13] "Even the most precedent-breaking New Deal projects reflected capitalist thinking and deferred to business sensibilities. Social Security was modeled, often irrelevantly, on private-insurance systems." [14]

The inclusion of private insurance principles in the Social Security Act lessened the burden of individual responsibility without departing from the traditional beliefs. Other portions of the Act, limited as they were to certain categories of needy persons, did not require such a rationalization; they were governmental "charity," whereas the general program became "insurance." In the United States, the typical American beliefs that business leaders could solve their problems without interference by outsiders delayed the acceptance of the new role of social welfare, and perhaps led inevitably to the strategy early in the Depression of stressing the fundamental soundness of the economy and ignoring the difficulties, hoping thereby to restore "confidence."

Procrastination in dealing with economic catastrophe had been evidenced on a smaller scale many times before. It was a natural outgrowth of traditional American views of economic "laws." Ignoring periods of economic decline and hoping that "confidence" would rectify the difficulties had become a standard response. Generally, the economy had been strong enough to recover without greatly increased governmental activity. This lent credence to the belief that no deliberate collective action was necessary in times of economic adversity. In Middletown, for example, both Chamber of Commerce and Rotary continually emphasized that the first duty of the citizen was to buy, and that "hopefulness" was the greatest prerequisite to the welfare of the nation. One businessman forecast a banner year, "because the people believe it will be, which amounts to the determination that it shall be. . . ." [15] The collapse of the economic structure in the 1930's, however, was so disastrous that it forced a wide acceptance of increased governmental activity, at least in connection with specific programs. The abstract question of governmental activity continued to cause uneasiness and, indeed, still often does.

It has been impossible to eliminate the belief that those who are not materially successful are necessarily lazy or weak. Even those shattered by the Depression often agreed with the valuation of the "possessors" and wondered whether the fault, after all, might be their own. This outlook has made a vulnerable target of "relief" for those who are disturbed by the retreat from the "ancient virtues." [16]

Sherwood Anderson travelled throughout the country during the early 1930's and interpreted its attitudes in *Puzzled America*. He says that hitch hikers nearly all began with an apology. "I've failed in this American scheme—It's my own fault" was the tone.[17] David Potter mentions that, even when access to economic advancement was lacking, Americans tended to see themselves as guilty and to blame themselves for not having achieved advancement. They had been taught to believe that "exemption from the negative impediments" was all that they needed, and they could not recognize that this exemption was meaningless in the absence of positive opportunity.[18]

Along with the tenacity of the belief in individual responsibility has come a steady growth in programs that are generally accepted even though they deny the validity of the belief. An official of the Social Security Administration writes that all other trends in public welfare over the last fifty years have been overshadowed by the development of an institutional mechanism for assuring a regular income to non-earning groups.[19] The passage of the Social Security Act was partially an attempt to reconcile a continued belief in individual responsibility with the acceptance of the inadequacies of the doctrine of individual sufficiency for modern society.

Since many of the traditional attitudes toward welfare measures survived the Great Depression barely shaken, it is not surprising that the people, prior to 1929, tended to overlook the evidence that showed their attitudes to be unrealistic. Investigations by state commissions throughout the 1920's produced results indicating that old age dependency was not limited to those who had been shiftless during their younger years,[20] but the results of these investigations seemed not to alter the stereotype held regarding persons on relief.

There were many indications even before the actual stock market crash that all was not well with the economy, and that the commonly held attitudes toward relief and other welfare measures were fast becoming less relevant to reality. In the later 1920's, community relief sources began to feel the pressure of unemployment. In Middletown, where the long slump of unemployment had begun as early as March 1924, the wife of a prominent businessman summed up what the Lynds believe to be the sentiment of the business class when she mentioned that persons often came to the house saying that they could not get work, but that she did not believe them because she believed that anyone who really tried could "get work of some kind." [21]

Though generally hidden by surface prosperity and the existence of various forms of relief programs at the community level, unemployment and other conditions requiring relief greatly increased in the late 1920's. Many social workers became alarmed at the problems of unemployment in the midst of prosperity. At the International Conference of Settlements in 1928, the Belgian economist Henri de Man declared that industrialism not only produces more goods, it also produces more unemployment. The National Federation of Settlements that same year found unemployment to be the "prime enemy of the American family." [22]

Pre-1929 welfare data do not exist either for entire cities or for the nation, but they do exist for some public welfare departments and for individual relief agencies. These show that during the prosperous twenties there was a uniformly rapid increase in relief costs.[23] Foreign observers have also noted the seriousness of the unemployment problem in the United States before the actual onset of depression and have mentioned that, despite the many new jobs and trades, the rise in population kept the number of jobs needed in excess of the number available.[24] This situation ran directly counter to the prevailing economic assumptions. Technological unemployment proved to be a much more serious force than had been anticipated and, except for the wartime boom and its aftermath, has continued to exceed expectations.

When major troubles are absent or hidden, the American generally has been little troubled about imbalances in the social structure. He typically has not concerned himself with difficulties that were not immediately apparent, and by and large he has failed to admit the existence of difficulties that he could not rationalize for consistency with his ideology. The traditional beliefs contained suspicion of governmental power even if exercised with the best of intentions. (This, of course, did not prevent the extensive *use* of governmental power.) Today, however, even the ideology often allows strong governmental action in the economic sphere if it is described with the vocabulary of free enterprise. Hence, the complicated nature of the programs through which the state generally acts.

When the United States was finally forced to adopt a program of social security, its mechanism took the form of a huge insurance plan, and so avoided the pitfalls that would have awaited a measure giving people "something for nothing" on so great a scale. Characteristically the symbol of the insurance company "allows us to live at peace with our ideals, and still support systematically a vast class of people." [25] There were other, much more realistic justifications advanced for the Act, it is true—many of them realistic by any standard. Only the "insurance-company model," however, gripped the minds and imaginations of the people. (See chapter III.)

Several New Deal scholars, without detracting from the importance of the Act as a social advance, have chronicled the complications introduced into the program by the American ideology. Leuchtenburg, for example, called the law "astonishingly inept and conservative" in many respects. He mentions that in no other of the world's welfare systems "did the state shirk all responsibility for old-age indigency and insist that funds be taken out of the current earnings of workers." He says that the accumulation of vast reserves and the use of regressive taxation "did untold economic mischief." Those who most needed coverage, farm and domestic workers, were excluded as were those whose lack of income was caused by illness.[26]

Some critics of the Act, at the time of its passage, believed that it posed an impossible bookkeeping task, but that the features responsible for this (those composing the "insurance company model") could be done away with gradually as the program got underway.[27] The bookkeeping task proved to be a great one, but one characterized more by size than by complexity. Developments in the mechanized processing of data, therefore, enabled the program to operate without eliminating the symbols. This is perhaps one reason for the great and enthusiastic acceptance of social security measures by the general public throughout the years. It has now become possible to speak of the exercise of governmental authority in terms hitherto reserved for private action.

Similarly, the Lynds found in their second study of Middletown that the existence of "predatory" business practices, the evident maldistribution of wealth, and the unreality of the idea of a universally accessible economic ladder did not damage the ideology. The citizens continued to justify their laissez-faire outlook by the existence of universal suffrage and the possibility of vertical economic mobility. Although they accepted governmental action as the nature of the situation required, they retained the belief in the "virtues" of self-help as opposed to the "immorality" inherent in many types of welfare measures.

The Lynds point out that dreams persist long after they have become anachronistic—indeed, into eras "bristling with palpably contradictory realities," if they reflect strong public desire.[28] This is especially true if the dreams are clothed in language seemingly consistent with reality.

Middletown reacted to the economic crisis similarly to other parts of the nation. Individual resourcefulness could not alone enable a factory worker to support himself and his family when he and hundreds of others were suddenly without jobs at a time when employment opportunities were lessening in virtually every kind of work. In the midst of this situation at the beginning of the thirties, the majority of the people retained their doctrines of self-reliance.[29] When Middletown's Central Labor Union or Rotary Club assembled in 1935, the members were much the same as in 1925, and were listening largely to the same speakers and the same ideas.[30]

Though this point may be exaggerated, it is significant. Despite the persistence of the old ideas, the city voted fifty-nine percent for Roosevelt in 1936. The Lynds admit that this is difficult to explain. They say that "radicalism" had made no inroads into the community, and that the people had not come to desire drastic change. They believe it likely that the voters simply recognized a vote for the New Deal as representing a possibility for improving personal security.[31] If the Lynds are correct in their observations that the people of Middletown retained their beliefs in the doctrines of individual responsibility and did not desire drastic change, yet voted for the New Deal in an effort to improve their personal security, it is apparent either that the New Deal was seen to be consistent with the ideology, or that the ideology, at least in this case, did not govern.

That the most significant social welfare measure of all, the

Social Security Act, ostensibly took the form of a gigantic insurance company, is evidence (regardless of European precedent) that form was as important as substance. On the practical
level the people accepted the measures necessary to relieve the
more severe of the economic problems. Conflict with the ideology resulted in rationalization, not in revision of the ideology.
The huge majorities supporting President Roosevelt in practice have often obscured the fact that much of the old ideological strains persisted in theory, or in the "American mind." Also,
as Commager points out, each student of the American mind
must consider that "thumping majorities" four times endorsed
the President, but must not fail to allow for the fact "that on
each occasion the majority of the wise, the rich, and the well-
born voted the other way." [32] The "wise, the rich, and the
well-born" no doubt contribute more to the shaping of the
American ideology than their numbers would indicate. The
generalization about the wealthy may have been much less applicable to the election of 1964, but the situation was more
complex than in 1936. Much of the landslide in favor of President Johnson seemed to have resulted from a negative reaction
to the personality or the image of his opponent. The elections
of 1960 and 1968 may be more indicative.

In his perceptive work *The Organization Man,* William
Whyte notes that few of the middle-class couples in his study
bother to save because so much now is being saved for them.
Significantly, they do not dwell upon social security but upon
the compulsory savings bestowed upon them by the organizations for which they work. He remarks that it produces discom-
fort for middle-class persons to dwell upon the benefits of welfare statism.[33] A certain anti-governmental attitude becomes
apparent when it is seen that compulsory governmental welfare
programs may produce uneasiness, but that compulsory corporate insurance and pension schemes do not.

The two studies of "Plainville," Missouri furnish material for
the study of the American ideology as manifested in a rural
area and a presumably representative village. The first study

took place in 1939–1940; the second in 1954–1955. These are especially interesting because they cover both the early stages of the programs under the Social Security Act, and the period after the greatly liberalizing amendments of 1950. According to the author of the second study, Art Gallaher, Jr., its purpose was to examine the "short-term processes of culture change, especially directed culture change." [34]

In Plainville just prior to World War II, no local recipients of government money were thought to be "earning their living," except for workers on WPA and NYA. Even being "one o' them WP-ers" carried a social stigma. Plainvillers criticized the WPA because it "made work" and because it hired men who, in their eyes, were worthless. On the other hand, they fully accepted the CCC, because, regardless of the class from which it recruited, it "built boys up" and "learnt 'em things." [35]

During the Depression, government agencies began almost exclusively to conduct charity activities that once were carried on primarily by churches, lodges, and neighbors. The people of Plainville used the government programs extensively, but "cussed" them incessantly for "ruining this country," for "meddling with business" and with "the way farmers know to do things," and for "making people unwilling to work and ruining people's characters." One resident remarked that if the New Deal had merely been instituted by Republicans, it would have been approved overwhelmingly; but, since it was a Democratic program, the strongly Republican community felt duty-bound to oppose it, even while taking full advantage of all its services. [36]

One of the principles most offensive to the citizens of Plainville was that of "cash without work." They did not question the distribution of food and other commodities to those in need since this resembled the familiar charity gifts from local sources. It is interesting that many critics of governmental health insurance in later years strongly opposed the distribution of a service (commodity) but approved the cash payments that had become a "firmly accepted principle." Their point is that the recipient is free to spend a cash supplement where he will, but has his freedom abridged if offered a service. The concern of these critics typically does not extend to the freedom of the indigent or the "medically indigent," however, since those who are in actual need, they believe, should receive service through the Medical Aid to the Aged, or Kerr-Mills, program.

The Plainville residents who were shocked at cash payments seem primarily to be reacting as classic rural American Anglo-Saxon Protestants to the changes involved in accepting a technically oriented money economy. Their concern was moral. Their ethic said that a man should work, and that to receive pay without work was wrong. Charity could be offered and accepted on humanitarian grounds, but the recipient was the object of pity. Many of the modern critics base their objections not upon morality, which can allow for humanitarian exceptions, but upon freedom, for which such exceptions are irrelevant. To establish a position based upon a support of freedom, but only for those who can afford it, was not a fault of Plainville society.

Though many of the traditional modes of thought remained, the Plainville of fifteen years later had seen many changes. The Plainville citizens of the middle 1950's were no longer so isolated, and many had grown up under welfare programs and governmental controls. The Plainville youth seemed to have developed economic attitudes fully in keeping with the money economy. Very few worked for the accumulation of land and surplus cash, as had previous generation; the major concern was their earning potential at any given time. Gallaher's description of the economic behavior of the young people of the town could have been a description of American youth in general written by any of several observers of the American scene. In justifying their preoccupation with the present, some of them, facetiously, says Gallaher, rationalize their unconcern for the future and for economic independence by saying that "the government will take care of you when you get old." [37]

The impact of government programs upon the community is undoubtedly very great. Gallaher mentions social security, GI training, military disability payments, civil service, and various other payments as well as the salaries of the administrators of government programs who live in the county. He quotes Plainvillers as saying, "there's a lot of people here living out of the post office," and says "it is estimated" (he does not say by whom) that over twenty percent of the total cash circulated in the county in 1954 came from federal sources.[38]

One of the greatest effects of the programs providing for old persons has been to remove their feelings of guilt that they are burdens upon their children and concomitantly to remove the obligation from children to care for their parents. Even though the payments tend to be extremely small, they help to give some measure of security. But regardless of the advantages, many Plainville citizens during the course of the second study expressed uneasiness regarding these programs. They believed that it was less "honorable" to depend upon the government than to earn a living for oneself. As a result, many of the most severe critics of the pensions under Old Age Assistance were those older persons who had been economic successes, and who resented seeing those who, in their eyes, had been poor workers receiving the same amount as those who had worked hard, but who had suffered misfortunes. A sense of social stigma sometimes caused pensioners to cash their checks outside the community.[39] The symbols surrounding payments under Old Age and Survivors' Insurance, however, enabled the "social security" program to avoid the opposition that met the "charity" programs, such as Old Age Assistance. The Plainvillers regarded social security as "earned" retirement, and therefore within the strictures of their beliefs.[40]

The citizens of Plainville, Missouri seem to be well within the stream of American thought in their newly-found concern with security. Max Lerner has said that, except for health matters, Americans of today are concerned about security most of all.[41] This includes those who are most afraid of "creeping socialism" and the "welfare state." Regardless of the party occupying power, they look to government for measures that once would have been considered revolutionary and "radical" but that now are believed to be consistent with the doctrines of individual responsibility. They also look to the "private sector," the labor unions and the corporations, for the welfare funds and other fringe benefits that have climbed relatively recently to a position of prominence in collective-bargaining efforts. The place of security in the American hierarchy of goals is a matter of record.

In 1953, Columbia University's American Assembly devoted its entire deliberations to the study of economic security for Americans. Its final report mentions that the participants had agreed, at the start of their discussions, that "a striving for security is part of the temper of our time." [42] In spite of the general retreat from risk and the constant concern with economic security, the suspicion that such a concern is degenerate persists. The ideology still holds that there is some antagonism between security and individual initiative, that quality upon which the free-enterprise system is often thought to be dependent. Much of this attitude is based upon an uncritical view of society. Galbraith points out that preoccupation of workers with old age pensions and unemployment insurance generally seems deplorable to business executives who would refuse to work for a company from which they could be discharged arbitrarily, or which did not furnish adequate retirement benefits. Entrepreneurs whose prices neither vary from those of their competitors nor fluctuate with market conditions, charge farmers with disloyalty to the free price system.[43] The fears of those who believe the search for security to be inimical to continued economic progress may have abated somewhat, but they have not been eliminated even when faced with the coincidence of economic growth and a general preoccupation with security.

the american process of rhetorical reconciliation

The practice of the rhetorical reconciliation helps to explain how American society escapes many of the strains that might be expected when its professed ideals conflict with many of its accepted practices. There is a tendency to describe accepted practices in ideologically acceptable terms, whether or not the terms are truly descriptive of the practices. Of course, this is unique neither to the United States nor to the twentieth century. Writers on language have noted similar linguistic practices since the early days of Western civilization. What is significant is the metamorphosis of the normal language shifts in American society into a rhetorical reconciliation between opposing practices and beliefs; a reconciliation that serves to perpetuate the conflict by rationalizing practices and delaying changes in ideology. Whether this is also the case in other countries is not at issue. The purpose here is to describe certain facets of American culture, not to prove its uniqueness.

Pareto may possibly have anticipated the notion of the rhetorical reconciliation in his theory of "residues" and "derivations." Without necessarily subscribing to his attempt at system building, one may readily applaud his description of imprecise thought and expression. "Residues" and "derivations" are opposed to "scientific" or "logico-experimental" thought. A residue, asserts Pareto, must not be confused with the sentiment or instinct to which it corresponds, but is the manifestation of that sentiment or instinct.[1] A derivation results from a residue and is sentiment in thinking. His elaborate classification of derivations includes "indefinite terms designating real things" and "indefinite things corresponding to terms," "terms with numbers of meanings, and different things designated by single terms"; and "vague, indefinite terms corresponding to nothing concrete." [2] He observes that people accept derivations not so much because they are convincing, but because they express "clearly ideas that people already have in a confused sort of way." [3]

Expressed more simply, all this seems to mean that thought is often imprecise, and that vague language is the result, and perhaps vice-versa. This is a beginning, but still does not adequately account for the development of the rhetorical reconciliation. The missing portion of the explanation may be found in the nature of a populous democratic society. Mannheim, in a perceptive passage, notes an inherent contradiction in a democratically organized society. Democracy mobilizes the energy of the individual, but also must find a way partially to neutralize that energy, since order is not possible if each person uses his energy to the fullest. There is a need, he believes, for devices involving "undemocratic or anti-democratic potentialities." These are not, however, imposed. They are the "voluntary renunciation by the mass of the full use of its energies." This natural tendency may become extreme and result in a "socially-induced stupidity" which permits "some organization or machinery" to think for the people. Thus American social science, says Mannheim, often tends to attempt to develop new knowledge without " 'thinking' about reality, relying solely upon routines of fact-finding, questionnaires, etc." [4]

The rhetorical reconciliation seems to be a similar expression of the willingness to forego thought—an outgrowth of usual linguistic and democratic tendencies. Universal literacy alone, therefore, in the absence of an education conducive to sound

methods of thought, may not enable the people to realize all
the benefits foreseen by its early advocates. Indeed, it may be
insufficient to sustain a modern democracy indefinitely with
proper regard for civil liberties and constructive action. The
education necessary for the survival of the modern democratic
state must prepare citizens to cope with a society that encour-
ages them to be gullible.[5]

Commager mentions the paradox of a society in which all
are literate but in which telegraph companies keep stocks of
"canned" messages to save patrons the trouble of devising their
own. He says that administrators, educators, and businessmen
have for so long used pieces of paper for real things that they
have come to believe that the abstractions are the real things.
He fears that this generation, for all its elaborate records,
knows less of human nature than did those that lacked forms
and questionnaires. Under these conditions language has become "artificial and derivative"; aided by the efforts of "advertisers, government bureaucrats, and schools of education,"
people have learned to say "simple things in complicated
ways." [6] Though this may be intemperate, there is enough
truth in it to warrant concern for the direction in which the
society is heading.

The non-economic role of advertising in a democracy is directly relevant here. There are considerable implications of
concern to the democratic theorist who recognizes the social
importance of advertising as an institution of great force that is
not responsible to society and is hardly susceptible to control.
It is significant that advertising, in Potter's words, tends "less to
provide the consumer with what he wants than to make him
like what he gets." A major function of advertising is to discourage critical thought. It tends "to minimize information and
maximize appeal," resulting in more standardization among
the products generally, but with greater efforts to differentiate
them psychologically, "in terms of slogan, package, or prestige." [7]

The role of advertising in modern society is uncomfortably

illustrative of the susceptibility to propagandistic manipulation that Mannheim notes in fully developed democracies.
When this tendency goes to its limit, as in the cult of the "leader," the principles of democracy have vanished altogether since
all political decisions are controlled from above.[8] The modern
methods of social control in America, however, differ from the
popular stereotype involving manipulation of the masses by
persons or small groups. Though there are elements of such
manipulation in the United States, many of the significant
social controls seem to arise from the people and to be accepted spontaneously. This is apparent in matters of religion and
personal conduct, as well as in politics.

Aldous Huxley correctly points out that the early supporters
of universal literacy and a free press foresaw only two possibilities, true propaganda and false propaganda, but that the
actual development has been a communication industry devoted neither to the true nor the false, but primarily to the
"unreal, the more or less totally irrelevant." [9] He need not
have limited his statement to the communication industry.

Huxley charges that enemies of freedom practice systematic
perversion of the resources of the language so that their victims
are forced to believe, think, and behave as they, the "mind-
manipulators," desire. He concludes that an education for freedom must include an education in the proper uses of language.[10] Improper language, in this context, would mean not
only the usages consciously encouraged by the "mind-manipu-
lators," political or commercial, but those that arise through
ignorance, carelessness, or the rhetorical reconciliation of contradictory practices and ideology.

George Orwell has written a remarkable essay, "Politics and
the English Language," in which he makes a forceful case for
his belief that language deteriorates not merely because of the
influence of individual writers but because of political and
economic conditions.[11] He says not only that language becomes
"ugly and inaccurate" because of foolish thoughts, but that
slovenliness of language makes it easier to entertain foolish

thoughts. This, combined with a tendency toward "compart-mentalized thought," or the consideration of one issue in iso-lation from others that are similar, may help explain the ability of the American to accept an inaccurate or irrelevant descrip-tion of his practices with no consciousness of the contradiction.

Orwell describes most modern English prose, especially po-litical writing, as being characterized by a "mixture of vague-ness and sheer incompetence," in which the writer is unable to express his meaning and inadvertently says something other than he intends, or is "almost indifferent" to whether he ex-presses a meaning or not. Perhaps encouraged by constant ex-posure to the media of mass communication, the modern speak-er or writer of expository prose often speaks or writes by building his sentences with stock phrases rather than with words. Certain subjects seem virtually to insure that the typical discussion will avoid original thought or expression. Orwell says, for example, that "fascism" now is meaningless except to signify something undesirable. "Democracy," "freedom," "so-cialism," "patriotic," "realistic," and "justice" now each have multiple and contradictory meanings, and cannot be defined adequately because of pressure from those who use the words in devious ways. Whether or not there is a conscious effort to prevent clarification as Orwell alleges, it is true that the words lend themselves to use by those who have private definitions but who allow or encourage their hearers to interpret them in a different manner. The word "extremism" is a salient example from the 1964 presidential compaign.

Orwell says that modern political speech and writing are largely a "defense of the indefensible." He mentions the British rule in India, the dropping of the atom bombs on Japan, and the Russian purges and deportations as things that can be de-fended, but only by arguments too brutal for most persons to accept, and which are inconsistent with the stated aims of po-litical parties. Political language must, therefore, he believes, "consist largely of euphemism, question-begging, and sheer cloudy vagueness."

My discussion of the uses of language does not extend to literary and artistic uses, but is limited to the role of language as the major instrument for the precise expression of thought. Neither does it accept the position of the semanticists, especially the popularizers of General Semantics, who at least by implication view language as a hindrance to thought, a distorting window between man and reality. Orwell mentions that Stuart Chase and others have almost claimed that all abstract words are meaningless, and have therefore advocated "a kind of political quietism." [12] One cannot struggle against fascism, for example, since no one knows what it is. Orwell says that it is unnecessary to accept such absurdities as this to recognize that the present situation of political confusion is related to the decay of language. Nevertheless, regardless of these and similar criticisms, works such as those of Chase can give valuable illustrations of the effects of the misuse of language, if they are used judiciously.

Ogden and Richards write that the most conservative force in our lives is the power of words.[13] This makes it all the more difficult to make an ideology based upon one set of conceptions consistent with conceptions built upon a different terminology. The difficulty is further increased if the original ideology has been formed without sufficiently contrasting it with other systems of values. This helps to explain the tendency to rationalize practices by imprecision in language, rather than by changing the ideology to make it consistent with the practices.

The European reformer could easily adopt socialism, since he had merely to adopt a language slightly more radical than that which he had used previously. For an American this generally has been impossible. In his discussion of this idea, Louis Hartz mentions that the language of Wilson was closer to the language of McKinley than to that of De Leon, and says that if anyone believes an economic boom to have been responsible, he need only to look at the New Deal. President Roosevelt eschewed the language of the European liberal reformers even when adopting many of their "quasi-collectivist" measures. He stressed his pragmatism, his solving of "problems," which, says Hartz, meant that New Dealers, like the Progressives before them, rarely drifted into socialism.[14] This can be overstated since many of the New Dealers, even upon occasion including the President, did introduce some innovation in language as well as in practice; but there is enough truth in the generalization to explain why the term "socialist" came largely to be accepted in this country as a synonym for "un-American" (itself a term devoid of meaning, but with emotional force) and why it retains this connotation.

The acceptance of symbols regardless of meaning is not unique to the United States, and has not progressed so far here as in some societies. Indeed, an acceptance of symbols is necessary to a degree for the preservation of a state and a well ordered social fabric, but the extent of this acceptance must be limited if the population is to be creative and independent.

The effect of an extreme public gullibility in the acceptance of symbols and the rejection of the rational has been amply illustrated during the last three decades. Jerome Frank, the lawyer, says that he thinks of what Hitler did to Germany when he reads Schopenhauer to the effect that:

> At the sound of certain words . . . the German's head begins to swim, and falling straight away into a kind of delirium, he launches into high flown phrases which have no meaning whatever. He takes the most remote and empty conceptions, and strings them together artificially, instead of fixing his eyes on the facts, and looking at things and relations as they really are.[15]

Fortunately, the symbols of the United States generally have not lent themselves to excesses, but an extreme acceptance of symbols can be dangerous regardless of the nature of the symbols themselves. Civil liberties and the Bill of Rights, for example, have upon occasion been assaulted in the name of "Americanism." Often in modern America citizens thoughtlessly repeat the familiar words of the Declaration of Independence or the Bill of Rights. Legislators recognize that the support that a pending bill can command is often more closely related to its viability as a symbol than to its actual provisions.[16] Consistent with this has been the change in name of the federal government's Bureau of Public Assistance to the Bureau of Family Services. Though the change was in name alone, officials remark in private conversation that it has "enhanced the Bureau's image in the field" and has made it easier to recruit qualified personnel.

An example of the strength of symbols to the American public, regardless of content, is the degree to which the use of the word "socialism" is divorced from reality. Social insurance, before its adoption, was advocated at least as consistently and forcefully by the Socialist Party as by any other, major or minor. Now, although extensions of the programs may still be labelled socialistic, social security is extolled by the general public and by both major parties. Federal officials often refer to the system as being all-American, or as American-as-apple-pie. Supporters of the system's expansion, such as J. Douglas Brown of Princeton, reiterate that social security is uniquely American, that it is the antithesis of socialism, and that it has been demonstrated to be "conservative" in principle.[17] In point of fact, however, Herman and Anne Somers, the perceptive students of social insurance and health economics, point out that Americans are pragmatists in behavior even though they are traditionalists in vocabulary, and they remark that their studies indicate that the differences between American social security and foreign systems are often exaggerated.[18] Any attacks upon the existing programs tend to concentrate upon actuarial soundness and whether social security actually is "insurance" or not. Responsible political elements now rarely, if ever, directly challenge its existence or underlying principles.

The American ideology consists primarily of broad generalities. It favors "democracy" and it abhors "socialism." Yet it seems inadequate to serve as a guide to specific actions. Generally, abstract terms are not readily thought of in terms of specific programs, and are judged against the ideology, while specific programs are judged mainly in terms of their expected effect. Hartmann's study of a Pennsylvania county discovered that many of the voters wanted specific measures that would fit into what he termed a socialistic program, but did not want them to be called socialistic. Almost two-thirds of those he polled would have denied teaching certificates to those who believe in socialism, whereas those same persons, according to Hartmann, "believe in what would, by every historical and economic criterion, have to be called socialistic proposals." [19]

He defined "radicalism" as advocating collectivism; for example, national ownership of resources and industries, as well as "internationalism" and social insurance; "conservatism" he defined as beliefs favorable to the preservation of the *status quo* (this was during the mid 1930's). He then assessed the agreement with "radical" propositions of groups ranging from those to whom the term "socialist" was most favorable to those to whom it was repugnant. The differences were slight. When he recalculated the averages, eliminating the responses to questions containing the word "socialism," all differences disappeared.

Though Hartmann's study has severe limitations (it is based upon a poll of 168 presumably "representative" citizens of Centre County, Pennsylvania) and the adequacy of his definitions is open to question, his findings are valuable if used with caution. Neither the Republican nor the Democratic parties, occupying respectively first and second place in strength in the county, advocated the policies implicitly advocated by the voters he questioned. The study demonstrates how words and symbols may lose and acquire meanings, but retain their effect upon the people. Hartmann concludes that those in the study apparently would prefer to have socialism introduced into the United States through the medium of the Republican Party.

The prevailing impersonal linguistic style, avoiding as it does the specific in favor of the vague and general, makes any analysis difficult. Often it completely masks an absence of thought. Because the language is so familiar, tautologies frequently sound quite meaningful. It would probably be incorrect to attribute the responsibility for this to any group. Certainly advertisers, politicians, and others have encouraged the tendency but it seems likely that they are merely reflecting the influence of their culture.[20]

Chase is probably correct when he maintains that semantic analysis helps explains many baffling contradictions.[21] Surely "fair-trade," "quality-stabilization," and "right-to-work" laws have gained much support that would not be theirs had it not been for the shrewd selection of adjectives. Throughout the commercial sphere, as well as the political, this usage obtains. "Special checking accounts," "revolving credit," and various "thrift plans" are often the means of charging the consumer more than he otherwise would pay for the same or similar services. The American Medical Association was extremely perceptive in basing its massive campaign in answer to President Truman's suggestions for national health insurance in the late 1940's upon the substitution of the term "socialism" for "insurance." John Kenneth Galbraith has called it a "workmanlike achievement in the technique of argument." [22]

Though political oratory in the United States and elsewhere rarely has been noted for precision and rationality, probably no period in American history has encouraged more empty and misleading rhetoric (speaking primarily of peacetime rhetoric) than the last few decades. To avoid the moral crisis that would have been the result of a frank adoption of programs that, though contrary to the ideology, were necessary to prevent the further breakdown of the social fabric, American society consciously or unconsciously adopted the rhetorical solution. "Clearly it was necessary to clothe ancient rights in modern garments, to supplement traditional freedoms adequate to the pastoral society of the eighteenth century with new ones efficacious in the industrial society of the twentieth." [23] The new developments were often described with language from an earlier time, which led the people to believe that truly new institutions are merely extensions of the old. Contributory social insurance illustrates this. It involved a new conception, so far as the major strains of American culture were concerned, and, for the first time, it enabled the public to accept the idea of governmental responsibility for those in need through some means other than "charity." Yet it was "insurance," requiring payments upon the part of the insured and basing his return upon his contributions, and it avoided "government interference in business." [24]

John Kenneth Galbraith has analyzed the situation and refers to the present as the "Age of the Wordfact." [25] The "wordfact," he says, replaces reality with words as a precise substitute. This brings the convenience of substituting for existence the mere statement that something exists. The public leader has only to find the language that will enhance the reality adequately, and he can transform the manifestation of anti-American sentiment abroad into the work of a "small number of Communists, acting under outside orders" or of a "misguided minority." The loss of the U-2, instead of a defeat, proved the weakness of opposing defenses; unemployment, far from being a curse, introduces a needed and desirable "slack" in the system (no properly run economy can be without it), and bad television programs are merely the "precious manifestation of the freedom of speech." Galbraith (in 1960) cited health care for the aged as a political issue upon which careers have been furthered by indicating an almost "uncontrollable desire" to enact legislation, rather than actually by passing laws.

One of the basic effects of the distortion of language, whether deliberate for purposes of a political gain or prestige (as in the case of the "wordfact") or simply accidental, is a tendency toward an isolation from reality. As is evident in the discussion of the Senate debates (see chapter VI), many of the attitudes toward social security expressed today display this tendency. Frequently both those who are critical of the program (or its extension) and those who are firm supporters tend to approach the question from the bias of the American ideology. Rather than accepting social insurance as a new function in society, they both tend to think of it in terms of the older social organizations. The "conservatives" tend to support the existing programs, but view them as increased governmental acceptance for relief, or as charity programs conducted in such a manner that there will be the least "threat to self-esteem and character" consistent with "the removal of responsibility for one's own future." The "liberals," on the other hand, often tend to think of the social insurance programs as nothing more than insurance. Few charges by conservatives draw more fire from liberals than those that social security is not "really" insurance. Many words have gone into the efforts to prove that the system is or is not "really" funded, or partially funded, and is or is not financed upon a "pay-as-you-go" basis. When certain elements have charged that "insurance" is a misnomer, the supporters of social security have feared attacks upon the fundamental principles of the system. Generally the charges have been attacks, but not all such assertions need be. Regardless of whether the term "insurance" (or the compromise "social insurance") is appropriate, the programs are in existence and have functioned effectively for more than a quarter of a century. Supporters who attempt to answer the charges of critics from the standpoint of the same bias as the critics suffer an inherent handicap.

Much discussion of social security in the United States, therefore, has been at a level divorced from reality because both supporters and detractors have tended to approach the subject with an ideological orientation that is inapplicable. In other words, the "conservatives" have often accepted social security as a modern substitute for philanthropy, whereas "liberals" have often spoken of it in the language used to describe an institution of private enterprise that "just happens" to be operated by the government. Both viewpoints are essentially humanitarian, both contain some truth, but neither is an appropriate view of a social institution which the American ideology renders fundamentally incapable of adequate description.

Imprecision in language discourages a spirit of analysis or interpretation and leads to unsound and often extreme infer-ences. Though such a tendency is painfully evident, a few examples will be valuable for purposes of illustration. To begin with, it is interesting to compare the attitudes of "conservatives" with those of the economist Friedrich A. Hayek regarding welfare measures. In *The Road to Serfdom,* Hayek says explicitly that an "extensive system of social services" is compatible with the preservation of competition if the system of services is properly organized.[26] He says that freedom is endangered only when a society attempts to provide its citizens with a given level of comfort, or attempts to insure the relative position enjoyed by a person or group when compared with others. Specifically mentioning sickness and accident, he says that, in the case of "genuinely insurable risks," there are strong arguments to support comprehensive systems of social insurance.[27]

The wide acceptance of Hayek's work by "conservatives" is, in view of these statements, frequently based more upon the symbols called to mind by the title than upon the contents. Daniel Bell points out that "liberals" have paid no more attention to the contents of the book than have the "conservatives," seeing in them only "stale Liberty League clichés." He concludes that no one actually wants economic liberalism, except as an ideology.[28]

A speech by former President Hoover in 1941, on "The Fifth Freedom," presents a succinct example of the effect of the use of cliches in leading thoughts and arguments afield from the basic premises.[29] President Hoover called for the "Fifth Freedom—economic freedom—without which none of the other four freedoms will be realized." "To be free," he said, "men must choose their jobs and callings, bargain for their own wages and salaries, save and provide by private property for their families and old age." The first criterion, freedom of occupational choice (no doubt within limitations), is certainly one element of the complicated conception of freedom. The next, collective bargaining (though Mr. Hoover did not mention "collective"), is somewhat less so, although still definitely an element, and the last, the "freedom" to provide "by private property" for one's family and old age, is virtually meaningless. Is private insurance "private property"? Are Pension plans? Is social security? And why is the notion of private property pertinent in the context at all, except as a stereotype? Here, the significant element is the notion of security, not private property or competition. It would seem that the emphasis upon security almost required the association with private property to make it more nearly consistent with the ideology.

Of course, the overwhelming majority of Americans had rejected Mr. Hoover and his programs. In accepting Franklin D. Roosevelt they recognized the necessity for action; they accepted much that was new, and sometimes heard the President and others describe the new programs with words and metaphors that were innovative and truly descriptive. On the other hand, when the people accepted Roosevelt as president, they accepted a man who, in his first inaugural address, placed the achievement of a balanced budget as one of the nation's most urgent needs, who used as justification in his message to Congress proposing the Tennessee Valley Authority that it would be a corporation "possessed of the flexibility and initiative of a private enterprise," and who recalled the passions of early America by equating economic oligarchies with political oligarchies and decrying, not merely profiteers, but "economic royalists."

In the "bitter and defiant" Madison Square Garden speech of October 31, 1936, he defended both Old-Age Benefits and Unemployment Compensation by referring to them as furnishing "insurance policies" with "premiums" paid by the worker and his employer. In response to allegations from some employers that the benefits would never materialize, he played upon xenophobic fears by saying that those who suggested such a thing "attack the integrity and honor of American Government itself" and that they "are already aliens to the spirit of American democracy. Let them emigrate and try their lot under some foreign flag in which they have more confidence," he said to applause, neatly turning back upon his critics the techniques that they had used against him. Thus, many of even the newest and most innovative actions were obscured by traditional political rhetoric. As when he associated the new freedoms "from" with the traditional American freedoms "of," Roosevelt emphasized the familiar while introducing change. His technique was to avoid ideological confrontation so far as possible by blurring the lines of conflict. This was a flexible, pragmatic approach but it could lead to such stratagems as requiring Raymond Moley to weave together two draft speeches, one on high tariffs and one on low.[30]

In March of 1963, *The Nation's Business,* published by the United States Chamber of Commerce, printed an interview with a man of science, Vannevar Bush, entitled, "We're Moving Deeper into Welfare State" (*sic*). This article illustrates that training in the sciences does not guarantee that the person so trained will carry a habit of precision in thought beyond his technical specialty. Yet, because of his training and position, he often speaks out as an authority upon a wide range of subjects, and is accepted as such by a substantial number of persons.

In response to a question regarding the present direction of our political thought, Dr. Bush refers to a significant conservative trend, but says that the long-term trend has been, since the founding of the republic, toward "centralization," a "pure democracy," and occasionally in the direction of a "socialistic state." With the exception of the trend toward centralization, the response is meaningless without an understanding of the sense in which Dr. Bush uses "pure democracy," and "socialistic state." Obviously, it is nonsense to speak of a trend toward pure democracy in any large modern state if the term is defined literally to mean the direct exercise of sovereignty by the people. Both terms have been used as epithets by the "radical right" and have achieved some degree of emotional content in the absence of precise definition. The statement as it stands either is an inadequate expression of the thought, indicates that the thought was simply an amalgam of handy clichés, or was intended to arouse a specific emotional response in the reader without a concomitant exercise of reason.

When asked whether federal intervention to solve a particular problem brings with it the risk of damage from federal control, he replies that "of course" it does, and cites federally administered medical care (which was not a serious political issue in the United States) as a system that would restrict the patient's free choice in selecting hospitalization and would limit the medical profession's vigor and independence. At no point does he rely upon more than the "wordfact" to support his position.

During the health-care controversy of 1961–62 the English writer, Graham Hutton, wrote articles, all of which were slight variations upon the same theme, for several American magazines. Without question, the most widely circulated was one entitled "America—Beware of the Welfare State," published, characteristically, in the *Reader's Digest* of October 1961. This was reprinted in quantity and supplied to many physicians for their waiting rooms with an added heading to the effect that the debate upon health care made the article important reading for each "thinking American." It stresses that one's physician urges him to read it carefully. Though these articles were not written by an American and ostensibly are treatments of the British system of health care, they are pertinent here because of their large American audience and their obvious purpose as weapons in an American political and social controversy.

Hutton's major points are the deleterious effects of welfare programs and their extreme cost. In one article he says that a program such as that adopted by the British would cost the United States $55 billion annually;[31] in another, the figure is "well over 100 billion dollars a year." [32]

Hutton's most interesting arguments are those concerning the costs of the "welfare state." He says that social services in the 1948 British budget "ran away" with 46 per cent, while national defense (and this was at a time when the nation was at peace and was rebuilding from a war) took "only 19 per cent." By 1950, the budget had increased from 12 billion to 18 billion, with "*two fifths* of this greatly increased sum" going to the "welfare state." He proceeds to decry inflation and the oppressive costs of the programs. To illustrate that the expenditures are unnecessary, he writes that the welfare state is still popular with the majority of the people even though they spend about half again as much upon alcohol and tobacco as for rent, more on smoking than upon the entire National Health Service plus all private health service, and more on games, betting, and entertainment than upon all education both state and private. He comments that this does not present the picture of a needy people.[33]

Neither does it present the picture of a people burdened beyond endurance by oppressive taxation for welfare services. The devotion to shocking language and emotionalism evidently prevented Hutton from recognizing that his illustration destroys one of his two major arguments.

Another article, "Insurance and Medicine—The Crossroads," written by E. B. Reed, M.D., appeared in *Best's Insurance News* for December 1961, and is noteworthy mainly for the desperation of its language. The author, in a glaring *non-sequitur,* concludes that since forty percent of the income of the nation is not subject to the social security tax, forty per cent of the people are excused from the tax! Furthermore, he says, demolishing his conclusion, only the first $4800 of the income of the "other sixty per cent" is taxed (this is in 1961) and the man making $100,000 annually pays the same rate as the one who makes only $4800. Dr. Reed's other points are that the "wily politician" has tampered with the social security programs to such an extent that it is a "national disgrace." He cites the addition of survivors' benefits and disability insurance as examples and says that it is impossible to identify the original Act. He calls the fundamental issue a "definite change to the left" in our political thought.

In view of the prevailing imprecision in the use of the language, it is little wonder that such contradictions in political discourse often remain undetected. Since meaning evaporates, it makes little difference whether the speaker is aware of the contradiction or not. The misuse of language, tending both to reflect and to encourage imprecision in thought, may be more readily evident in political as opposed to non-political expression, but the difference is slight. Many writings in the social sciences, for example, make full use of clichés and the technique of the "wordfact."

Hans Zetterberg could well have used the conception of the "wordfact" in his description of one of the techniques that exists to ensure the appearance of "progress" in theoretical and applied sociology, when he remarks that in both the tendency is to substitute a change in technical vocabulary each decade for progress.[34] He says that the vocabulary of the social theorist of 1960 would be almost incomprehensible to the social theorist of 1930, and that the professional language of 1960 could not convey a description of current social practice to a social worker of 1930; yet the actual knowledge of the theorists and actual actions of the practioners are very likely identical.

In general, both "conservative" and "liberal" politicians shape their arguments around the same ideological symbols. This may partially be based upon expedience (the necessity to appeal to the public) but no doubt arises also from firm conviction. The significance is not merely that they use the same symbols to justify opposing positions, but that they both tend to see the same major symbols as keys to a particular issue, regardless of their actual relevance. Part of the difficulty of extending social welfare measures in this country has been caused by the tendency for both supporters and opponents to accept many of the symbols and biases that are contrary to the principles underlying the measures. This is required if both sides are to appear to be within the "American tradition," meaning that they are adherents to the American ideology; but it weakens the arguments of the proponents, who are forced to agree with their antagonists on many fundamental issues.

Though the basic acceptance of the key importance of the same symbols by both supporters and opponents undoubtedly has hampered the extension of the social security programs and the adoption of other related measures, it is likely that it makes each development more durable than if the symbols did not appeal to both sides. To gain acceptance, a new program must generally be described in terms consistent with the ideology shared by both parties, regardless of the substance of the program or the relevance of the terms. To an extent, therefore, the American ideology continues to aid the society, even in the mid-twentieth century. The consensus produced by its common acceptance has tended to prevent sharp polarities in political thought, and to some degree has modified political action. The ideology does not direct action, but the linguistic reconciliation of resulting measures with the ideology has certainly increased the public's acceptance of the newer programs.

The pragmatism that has enabled the culture to have its ideological cake and eat it too, has shielded it from the strains inherent in revisions of ideologies, and yet has permitted it to function effectively in situations that could not have been met by actions guided by the ideology. The American adherence to an ideology that bears little relation to practice, though it has been an effective accommodation to the complexities of the modern world, yet contains definite dangers. Alfred North Whitehead has said that "those societies which cannot combine reverence to their symbols with freedom of revision must ultimately decay, either from anarchy or from the slow atrophy of a life stifled by useless shadows." [35]

There has been a steady improvement over the last few decades, and there is considerable evidence that the future of democratic principles in American culture is bright. Nevertheless, the same flexibility that has enabled Americans to accept social security while retaining an ideology that would seem to require its rejection has enabled them to permit such things as the relocation of the Japanese-Americans during World War II, and the various governmental activities directed toward the ferreting out of undefined "un-American activities." All actions of this kind violate the rights of the individual in contradiction of a cardinal tenet of the American ideology. In the absence of a sound liberal education placing proper stress upon the role and effect of language, there is no guarantee that the finer traditions paid homage in the United States such as political democracy, civil and political liberties, and the importance of the individual can be adequately safeguarded.

the social security act
and the insurance-company model

The term "social security" refers to a number of things. In its broadest sense, it encompasses all social welfare measures; in its strictest sense, it can mean the variety of specific programs authorized by the Social Security Act. For most Americans, however, the term means the contributory social insurance programs—the familiar Old-Age, Survivors', and Disability Insurance, and, in later years, the "Medicare" program. It was partly in response to this narrower construction in the popular mind that the Social Security Administration was reorganized on January 28, 1963 to administer only these provisions of the Act. The categorical assistance programs are no longer administered by the Social Security Administration but by separate agencies of the Department of Health, Education, and Welfare. Other programs, of course, continue to be handled by the Department of Labor. For purposes of simplicity, the term "social security" is used in its popular sense throughout this study, except where the context clearly indicates another meaning.

There was a period exceeding a half century between the establishment of the world's first modern social welfare system —that begun in 1883 in Germany under Bismarck—and the passage of the American Social Security Act in 1935. Though it seemingly required the Great Depression to force the United

States to adopt a formal program of social security at the national level, the roots of the Social Security Act may be traced at least as far back as the 1909 White House Conference on Care of Dependent Children. This conference gave impetus to the idea of governmental pensions or allowances to widows with dependent children. Indeed, in *Agrarian Justice* written over a century earlier, Thomas Paine outlined a scheme that was similar in principle to social security, yet the same ideas sounded "radical" when proposed by such American pioneers of social insurance as I. M. Rubinow, Paul Douglas, and Abraham Epstein during the first three decades of the twentieth century.

The first of the mothers' pension plans was established in Denver, under the leadership of Gertrude Vaile, who had been active in the Charity Organization Society movement, and who was a student and friend of one of its noted leaders, Mary Richmond. In 1914, writing in Paul Kellogg's magazine of social reform, *The Survey,* she outlined the problems facing those who would lead the way to the establishment of similar programs. The difficulties, including apathy, were great and only meager results could be expected. A considerable number of state legislatures did pass some form of legislation, but many such laws did no more than authorize localities to set up programs if they chose.[1]

During the years following the White House Conference in 1909, numerous progressive associations and groups were bringing together social workers, such as Jane Addams and Grace and Edith Abbott, and influential figures such as Eleanor Roosevelt, Newton D. Baker, Louis Brandeis, and the prominent University of Wisconsin economist John R. Commons, who used their prestige to encourage reform efforts. Florence Kelley's National Consumers' League was one of the most militant of these organizations. Another, the Women's Trade Union League, fought long and hard against exploitation of industrial workers. The American Association for Labor Legislation, headed throughout its existence by John B. Andrews and his wife, grew from about two hundred members in 1906 to more than three thousand in 1919, and through writing and lobbying was instrumental in bringing about the adoption of rudimentary workmen's compensation laws in many states. Andrews was a student of John R. Commons and cooperated with him in several studies. He exerted great influence on many other reform groups.[2]

In 1913, the theoretical justification for the Social Security Act of 1935 was set forth in I. M. Rubinow's classic work *Social Insurance*. Rubinow was a physician turned economist and statistician. He had been with the U. S. Bureau of Labor and was a lecturer on social insurance at the New York School of Philanthropy. His book sets forth the idea of social insurance, traces its background and development in Europe, and explains the varying types then in existence. The publication of this volume marked its author as the pioneer authority on social insurance in the United States. Until his death shortly after the passage of the Social Security Act, he remained one of the foremost of a small group of American experts in the field. The final program owed much to his early and continuing efforts.

Rubinow pointed out the falsity of the argument that the high standard of American wages eliminated the need for social insurance. He said that wages were not sufficiently high to yield a continuous surplus and that an annual surplus of income was an unusual phenomenon in the working classes.[3] It required the severity of the Great Depression finally to produce action along the line Rubinow suggested.

During the rise of the progressive movement, social reformers developed a spirit of cooperation with many government officials at all levels. The social reformers considered the defeat of Theodore Roosevelt in 1912 to be a severe blow to their cause. Nevertheless, the cooperation continued to a certain extent during the Wilson Administration, but World War I destroyed it by redirecting popular concern and associating many reform programs with "pro-German" sympathies. It was impossible to restore the relationship during the era of "normalcy" after the war. The mood of the 1920's was far from conducive to reform measures.[4]

The first brief flurry of activity in support of governmental health insurance in the United States spanned the war years. In 1912, the American Association for Labor Legislation formed the nation's first Committee on Social Insurance. In 1913, the Association sponsored a national conference on social security which led to the drafting of a model social insurance bill, including health insurance provisions, for introduction into state legislatures. The Committee on Social Insurance appointed a subcommittee in 1914 specifically to prepare the bill, and the subcommittee completed its task in 1915. In the same year, the American Medical Association also evidenced interest in compulsory governmental health insurance, and formed its own Social Insurance Committee. Three of its members, Alexander Lambert, I. M. Rubinow, and S. S. Goldwater, all physicians, were members of the committee earlier formed by the American Association for Labor Legislation. Though the two associations were prepared to cooperate upon the medical issues involved, the period of cooperation was brief. By 1918, not only had serious opposition developed within the American Medical Association, but many insurance companies and pharmaceutical houses had also begun to work against the program.[5]

The model social insurance bill was introduced into the New York Legislature in 1916, 1917, and 1918; during these years, many legislatures established commissions to investigate the issues involved, the strongest ones being in New York and California.[6] The movement was furthered by a new book by I. M. Rubinow in 1916, *Standards of Health Insurance*.[7] In 1919, the bill providing for health insurance passed the New York Senate, but, even with the support of Governor Al Smith, it failed in the Assembly's Rules Committee.[8] By 1920, health insurance had ceased to be a serious political issue in the United States, and the American Medical Association went on record with a policy of strenuous opposition that lasted for more than four decades.

In August 1921, during the brief postwar depression that had begun in 1920, President Warren G. Harding called a Conference on Unemployment. The conference accomplished little, but the pressures on the participants had lessened because economic conditions had already begun to improve. The general attitude can be assessed by the response of Otto T. Mallery, chairman of the conference's Subcommittee on Public Works, to reformers' attacks upon the conference for not considering the idea of unemployment insurance. He said that for the conference to have considered an untried measure having no public support would have jeopardized serious discussion of other relevant issues. He was undoubtedly correct in supposing that to most Americans at that time the idea of unemployment insurance would have seemed outlandish.[9]

There was some talk, occasioned by the depression, of public works and centralized employment services, but the rapid economic recovery quickly stifled such notions. Likewise, when Paul H. Douglas, the University of Chicago economist and future United States Senator, published his *Wages and the Family* in 1925,[10] his suggestions that the United States attempt a program providing something similar to the family allowances already widely prevalent in Europe aroused little interest.[11] In many instances, proposals for social-security legislation brought expressions of horror. A Massachusetts study branded old-age pensions as 'a counsel of despair'. "If such a scheme be defensible or excusable in this country, then the whole economic and social system is a failure," it said.[12]

Despite the general mood of apathy toward social welfare during the 1920's, the spark of social reform did not die completely. The Fraternal Order of Eagles and the American Association for Labor Legislation jointly proposed that states adopt old-age pension plans, and drafted a model bill.[13] Paul Douglas writes that there were "certain undercurrents of public opinion which were beginning to change on the subject of old age pensions," even before the depression.[14] This is indicated by the fact that eight states had passed enabling acts permitting counties to set up pensions; of these states, Wisconsin and Minnesota provided for state aid to any county that did so.[15]

Anti-governmental attitudes, however, rendered extremely difficult the progress of any social legislation. Julia C. Lathrop, then Chief of the Children's Bureau (which was at that time in the Department of Labor), was astonished by "the popular distaste for governmental activity" in reaction to a proposed child labor amendment.[16] Similarly, Ethel Smith, chief lobbyist for the Women's Trade Union League, concluded in a report to the organization's board of directors in 1925 that opposition to the amendment "constituted opposition to any effective regulation, local, state, or national." [17]

Dr. Rubinow noted in 1926 that, despite rising wages, there was a rising social service case load occasioned by increasing unemployment. He called for social workers to turn from their preoccupation with "bad physical heredity, inadequate personality, lack of initiative, psychoses and neuroses, and constitutional inferiority . . . and take up the cause of social insurance." There was evidently little response.

The social historian, Clarke Chambers, notes that in the meantime others, particularly settlement workers, had become aware of the danger signals. In the winter of 1928, residents at the Chicago Commons began to report growing unemployment. Similar reports began to come from other settlements, but very few persons paid heed.

It was at this time, in 1927, that Abraham Epstein, the research director for the Pennsylvania Old Age Pension Commission, was instrumental in forming a new organization, the American Association for Old Age Security. Through his lobbying activities and publications, Epstein soon became one of the most prominent advocates of social insurance in the United States, along with others such as Paul Douglas and I. M. Rubinow. In 1928 he complained of a lack of zeal among welfare workers, charging that many of them were more concerned with means than with ends, and evidenced spirit only "during the annual 'zip-zip' community chest drives for funds." That same year, *Harper's Magazine* rejected one of his articles because of its allegedly "Bolshevik air"; but, at the same time, he began to notice more enthusiasm: not only were more countries adopting old age pensions, but his lecture audiences began to increase.[18] In 1931, largely because of depression conditions, his organization suddenly found itself influential.[19] In 1933, Epstein changed its name to the American Association for Social Security, reflecting the broadened interests of his group.

Early in the 1930's three books were published that added considerable impetus to the social insurance movement: Paul Douglas' *The Problem of Unemployment* (1931), Epstein's *Insecurity: A Challenge to America* (1933; revised 1936), and Rubinow's *Quest for Security* (1934).

Epstein wrote of social insurance as carrying the principle of private insurance "to its logical limit." [20] In considering the question of "compulsion," he granted that the word was offensive to many persons but argued that "compulsive legislation" was not new to the United States, and sometimes is a necessity.[21] He characterized social insurance as a "stabilizer" of the social order, and in discussing financing asserted that "income and inheritances taxes for the purpose of social insurance are equitable from every point of view." [22]

Rubinow's *Quest for Security* was the logical extension of his earlier work, *Social Insurance* (1913) —the first comprehensive treatment of the project in the United States. *Quest for Security* was an incisive analysis of the confused, illogical state of mind of most Americans on the subject of "relief." Why should accepting relief be a disgrace, he asked, when no one minds taking advantage of free concerts, regardless of whether they are financed by some patron of the arts or by the city. Social workers administering relief occasionally saw clients who possessed such pride that they refused material assistance. In such situations, he noted, the social workers used strong arguments to break down the client's "dignity" ("why should your family suffer because of your pride?") but secretly admired it. He cited studies showing that during early years of the Great Depression a "respectable non-pauperized family" typically endured from six to eight months of unemployment before applying for relief of any sort, public or private. Rubinow considered this to be "evidence of the moral strength of the masses, who will not seek help until in a desperate condition." [23]

With the assumption of the Presidency by Franklin D. Roosevelt in 1933, the hesitation came to an end. Two of the federal officials who were to be most influential in the government's attempts to provide social security were Harry Hopkins, the Federal Emergency Relief Administrator, and Secretary of Labor Frances Perkins, both of whom had long experience in social reform movements, the settlement houses, and the field of social work. Miss Perkins had been with Jane Addams at Hull House, had studied economics under Simon Patton (the noted University of Pennsylvania economist who boldly advocated governmental economic planning), had been executive secretary of the Consumer's League in New York, and had long been within the "inner circle" of the social work profession.[24] She also had travelled to England in 1931 at the request of Roosevelt, who was then governor of New York, to study the British system of unemployment insurance.[25] Hopkins had worked at Christadora House, a settlement in New York, and was a past president of the American Association of Social Workers.[26]

On June 29, 1934, the President issued Executive Order 6757 creating the Committee on Economic Security composed of the Secretary of Labor (Chairman), the Secretary of the Treasury, the Attorney General, the Secretary of Agriculture, and the Federal Emergency Relief Administrator. The previous day, the Attorney General had ruled that the National Industrial Recovery Act had empowered the President to create such a committee. Thus, President Roosevelt took concrete steps toward the creation of a system of social insurance which he had emphasized as a pressing need in his special message to Congress on June 8. The Committee's report, dated January 15, 1935, contained the outline of what was to become the social security system, and incorporated some of the principles of private insurance (or, as it will be called here, the "insurance-company model") into the provisions for Old-Age Benefits.

The Committee's recommendations were introduced into Congress in January by Representatives David J. Lewis (D-Md.) and Robert L. Doughton (D-N.C.) in the House, and Senator Robert F. Wagner (D-N.Y.) in the Senate. Though Representative Doughton (chairman of the Ways and Means Committee) had not previously been noted for support of social insurance, his bill (H.R. 4120) took precedence in the House. At this stage in the proceedings, the bill was called the Economic Security Bill, but the House Ways and Means Committee rewrote it extensively, and substituted its own bill (H.R. 7260). Thereafter it was referred to as the Social Security Bill, and it was this bill that the House passed and sent to the Senate Finance Committee, which reported it (and not the Wagner Bill) to the Senate for passage.[27]

Though the example of the private insurance company was certainly not the only argument used by proponents of the Social Security Bill, and applied only to one of its benefits, it was among their most forceful arguments and seemed certainly to have the greatest impact upon the public. The idea of incorporating the principles of private insurance, such as "premiums," certain provisions for individual equity, etc., into a social insurance system did not originate in the United States. In fact, though the program was described as "peculiarly American," the framers of the bill drew directly upon European precedent, dating from 1883 in Germany. Today the majority of the world's programs rely upon the "insurance concept." [28] Nevertheless, the deciding criterion of form seemed to be dictated more by American affection for private enterprise than by precedent; so nearly as can now be determined, no one seriously even proposed an alternative to the insurance-company model. It is significant that, under its provisions, the Committee, the Congress, and evidently the people of the United States were willing to postpone benefits for years after taxes began, to enable the program to be contributory and self-financing. This, of course, applies only to the general program, that of Old-Age Benefits. The programs that were limited to special categories (such as Aid to the Blind, or Aid to Dependent Children) , or that involved means tests were unaffected by the notion of insurance. A program applicable to the general population, however, seemed to require a rationalization ("old age" in this sense is not a special category, since the population generally can anticipate arriving at such a status) .

Congress seemed to be even more insistent upon the insurance-company model for this program than were the original planners. Both the Administration and the Congress were anxious to avoid contributions to Old-Age Benefits from the general revenues as had been contemplated in the original draft. Accordingly, the tax rates finally voted to finance the program were higher than those recommended in the report of the Committee on Economic Security.[29]

The original Act of 1935 provided for a rebate to those who had paid taxes but did not qualify for benefits. The Act did not provide for benefits until January 1, 1942, but the benefit formula was revised in 1939 and the original provisions were never put in force. They are of interest, nonetheless, because of their emphasis upon individual equity. Under the rebate arrangement, no one was to pay more into the system than he withdrew from it. It is apparent that the teachings of Epstein and Rubinow affected the Act in many respects. Both men believed in the insurance principle and both were students of European systems, most of which were built upon the principle.

Rubinow's discussion of his preference for contributory, as opposed to non-contributory, programs is especially illuminating. He maintained that a contributory program is more dignified, more "scientific," and eliminates the objection to pension schemes as thinly disguised "relief." Contributory programs also make it necessary to establish recipients' need and lack of resources, and are free from the even more objectionable inquiries into available means. Moreover, contributory programs do not have the "demoralizing influence" upon individual thrift of a straight pension based on need, because the means of the recipient would not affect his eligibility. He believed that contributory programs are sufficiently flexible to recognize differences in individual economic strata, and are appropriate for the needs of salaried classes for whom straight pensions offer too low a level of benefits.[30]

Other features of the 1935 act—ironically those that strengthen the insurance symbol—run counter to the teachings of Rubinow and Epstein. Both considered it an obligation of the government to contribute from general revenues to the old-age insurance system as part of the overall effort to foster the welfare of the people. Epstein, in fact, though applauding the act as a great step forward, strongly attacked its method of financing Old-Age Benefits. He charged that it was fiscally unsound, that the large trust fund would be dangerous, would invite "tampering," and would lessen purchasing power. He would have preferred some contribution from general revenues to reduce the amount of money withheld from circulation and to relieve the burden on wage earners.[31]

Many features combine to make up the "insurance-company model" that characterizes the system. Foremost among these are highly detailed record-keeping on an individual basis, the requirement that there be payments into the system (similar, at any rate in the popular imagination, to "premiums") by the citizen, and the avoidance of financing from general revenues. With its "insurance" emphasis and the efforts to portray the government as merely a "manager," not a participant, the scheme so carefully rationalized a governmental program in terms of a private-enterprise ideology that it effectively counter-

acted criticisms based upon the complexities of the arrange-
ments and the regressive nature of the taxation supporting
them.

The planners of the social security system, probably condi-
tioned by the traditional antipathy toward governmental involvement in social welfare, saw only two alternatives: either
some non-contributory program with means tests, or some sort
of contributory program without them. Other possibilities were
apparently inconceivable. In fairness one must grant that the
theoretical foundations of the Social Security Act may have reflected a true spirit of innovation that has become difficult to
recognize as such more than three decades later, yet an analysis
of the arguments for and against the Act in terms of their
relationship to American thought and experience suggests that
the program was simply an attempt to apply familiar, comfortable ideas concerning social welfare to a larger proportion of
the population. As Schlesinger notes, it seems probable that the
notion that private insurance should serve as the model was too
compelling.[32]

In formulating recommendations for an old age security program for the United States, the Committee on Economic Security reported that popular discussion of programs designed to
assure a measure of economic security to the aged distinguished
between non-contributory old age assistance and contributory
old age insurance. "It seems apparent, however, that an effective old age security program for this country involves not a
choice between assistance and insurance but a combination of
the two."[33] The committee defined "assistance" as a non-
contributory system based on need, "insurance" as a contributory system based upon a right to benefits regardless of need,
and "combination" as two separate systems operating simultaneously rather than a single system incorporating certain
features of both. Such a combination, in fact, exists at the
present time.

Regardless of the merits of the existing combination, it seems obvious that the two systems do not constitute the only viable possibilities. For example, the Committee might well have considered—but did not—the merits of some non-contributory system based not on need but on a right of every citizen to certain benefits merely by virtue of the fact of citizenship. However, a dominant ideology precluded this alternative by its general premise that an economic right arises from individual economic endeavor. This premise is not absolute since it would seem not to deny economic right based upon inheritance, but it seems safe to assume that it was at least influential in preventing the Committee from considering seriously many alternatives to the two it proposed.

In praising insurance systems, whether governmental or industrial, the committee stressed regularity of payment and freedom from means tests. These two factors, especially the latter, became the major arguments for a system based upon insurance principles. Though these factors are characteristic of such a system, an insurance scheme is by no means the only one that could incorporate them. The Committee may have examined other methods of providing freedom from means tests and discarded them in favor of the insurance approach, but its reports do not indicate this. Since the traditional role of the American government in social welfare had been based on charity, or providing assistance to those whose needs were great and who had no resources, the committee seemed unable to conceive an active role for the government that involved the payment of benefits as a right, except through the "insurance company" system.

In Europe the insurance mechanism predominated because the pioneering German and Austrian social insurance schemes, in the time of Bismarck, had incorporated into a compulsory governmental system the private and voluntary plans upon which they had been based. In the United States, on the other hand, the governmental system was a sharp break with the American tradition that opposed such action by the government. The insurance principle was so compatible with American thought and practice, however, that it seems no one seriously considered not following the European precedent.

Not all features of the program are consistent with the insurance-company model, though it remains dominant. As one example, the emphasis upon individual equity has steadily lessened. Moreover, there were elements even in the early program that were designed specifically for social purposes at the expense of individual equity. Low-income and short-term workers, for instance, received benefits in excess of those that would have been provided by a strict program of individual equity.

The revisions to the program in 1939 provided both major additions and definite changes in the principles of the system. This was the year in which survivors' benefits were added, giving not only a new benefit, but also an emphasis upon the family. This family emphasis, coupled with the elimination of the rebate, greatly weakened the principle of individual equity. From this point on, married workers, especially those with children, received much more for their contributions than childless or non-married workers. The low-income and short-term workers' advantages also increased. Nevertheless the public still tends to think of the program in terms of private insurance.

THE POLITICAL PARTIES

The social security system was a major subject of debate in the 1936 presidential campaign. The Prohibition Party claimed in its platform that it had been the very first party to endorse this idea of old age pensions, and it called for additional government aid to the elderly and the disabled.[34] Father Coughlin's Union Party platform called for security for the aged, charging that they had been "victimized and exploited by an unjust economic system which has so concentrated wealth in the hands of a few that it has impoverished great masses of our people." The Socialist Party favored immediate appropriation of six billion dollars for the relief of the unemployed for the coming year. To this they added support for unemployment insurance, old age pensions for all over sixty (to be financed through income and inheritance taxes as in the Frazier–Lundeen Bill) and health care for all to be provided "as a social duty, not as a private or public charity." The platform of the Communist Party contained an entire section entitled "Provide Unemployment Insurance, Old Age Pensions, and Social Security for All." The Communists defined social security in a broad sense, advocating the addition of health and maternity benefits.

The Democratic Party boasted of the Social Security Act and the measures it provided, and pledged to use it as a base to erect a "structure of economic security" for everyone. The Republicans, on the other hand, declared in their platform that real security would be possible only when the nation's productive capacity was sufficient to provide it and that, to attain that goal, they looked "to the energy, self-reliance and character" of the people, and to the system of free enterprise. Following this, however, they proposed a system for old age security built upon four parts: First, a pay-as-you-go system requiring each generation to support the aged and to determine "what is just and adequate"; second, a supplementary payment sufficient to provide income large enough to protect from want all American citizens over sixty-five; third, graduated payments to states and territories for cooperative financing of security programs that have met "simple and general minimum standards"; and fourth, "a direct tax widely distributed" to finance the federal portion of the program. The platform declared that this would be "consistent with sound fiscal policy" and would require contributions from all, since all would be benefited. The Republicans charged that the Social Security Act was unworkable because of administrative complexity, that its tax burdens would be great, and that it provided benefits to too few people.

The Republican proposals met with great favor from many

supporters of social insurance, notably those who had been disappointed with the terms of the Social Security Act. An editorial in *The Nation* of June 24, 1936, said that although "a direct tax widely distributed" sounded suspiciously as if it meant a sales tax, the social insurance plank of the Republican platform was in advance of the position of the Democratic Party in preferring social insurance revenue to be derived from general taxation.

In a letter to the editor published July 11, Evelyn M. Burns, then on the Economics faculty at Columbia University and vice-president of the American Association for Social Security, wrote that she was "very surprised" to read the editorial, since the Republican platform did not provide for social insurance at all as the phrase was generally understood. She pointed out that the platform did not mention benefits as a matter of right, but only on the basis of need. She agreed that the approach based on need did have a place in a social security program, that it was "complementary" and had already been provided by the Social Security Act as Old-Age Assistance. She added that the social security plan, regardless of the merits of its financing, did return at least something to the contributor, whereas the plan advanced by the Republicans would tax everyone but pay benefits only to those who subjected themselves to a means test. Further, the Republican plan would pay no benefits at all in states that might happen not to participate in the program. It is interesting to note that virtually the same arguments on both sides were duplicated in the Medicare controversy.

The editors hastened to reply that they had not meant to contrast the "illiberal Republican plank with the Social Security Act, but with the party's complete silence on the subject in 1932" and that they agreed completely with Mrs. Burns' statements, having written as they had "largely because of the reactionary nature of the [Republican] platform as a whole." The editors could as easily have contrasted the 1936 platform of the Democrats with that of 1932. The only parties that had specifically advocated social security measures in their 1932 platforms were the Farmer-Labor and the Socialist parties. Both had supported social insurance for many years, the Farmer-Labor Party since 1920, and the Socialist Party in every presidential campaign since 1900.

Though many minor parties had advocated social insurance, the closest the idea came to acceptance by a major party, before the days of Franklin D. Roosevelt, was its inclusion in Theodore Roosevelt's Progressive Party platform of 1912. Not until 1936 was the issue considered in the platforms of the Democrats and the Republicans. The only earlier mention of a related subject by the Democrats appears to have been in their platform of 1916, in which they supported a law providing for "the retirement of superannuated and disabled civil servants" so that "a higher standard of efficiency may be maintained." The Republicans' record was similar. Their only mention of a related subject before 1936 seems to have been in their 1924 platform, in which they called for the creation of a cabinet post of education and relief, to coordinate the various departments administering the federal government's "numerous and important" welfare activities.

The history of the political parties' positions on social insurance is a classic illustration of the validity of the contention that the major parties tend to be steadying, conservative influences, while the minor parties tend to develop or accept new ideas. The minor parties introduce new ideas into the actual realm of politics, where they are proved and either discarded or molded into relatively acceptable forms. After reaching this point, the major parties take over the ideas as their own, relaxing their conservatism enough to experiment with them only after they have been seasoned for years as the rallying points of minor parties and non-political reform movements. The major parties adopt innovations in many instances only after the activities of the minority parties and groups have made them, and the language used to describe them, politically "respectable."

Some of the more liberal thinkers, including some notable advocates of social insurance, refused to accept the Democratic platform of 1936 as more than a deception. The editors of *The Nation,* for example, in addition to their earlier expression of pleasure for the Republican platform, said in an editorial on July 4, 1936 that if they had not been familiar with the details of the "cumbersome, inadequate Social Security Act, with its vicious system of reserves which at best will provide protection for less than half of the unemployed and on a federal basis for scarcely a third of the aged, the Democratic pledge to provide economic security for all might be inspiring." Obviously, however, the rise of the image of the Democratic Party as the "Party of the Common Man" indicated that most Americans viewed the party much less critically than did the editors of the *The Nation.*

The general acceptance of the social security plan by the public prevented both parties officially from attacking the fundamental principle of governmental responsibility for the welfare of the people. Since the Democrats had passed the Act, the Republicans severely criticized it, but not its basic justification. Referring to social insurance, Governor Landon in a radio interview on May 7, 1936, said, "I'm for it. Every big industrial nation has had to move in that direction. In America we could once handle the problem pretty well by depending on individual thrift, family aid, local taxation and private contributions. These still have their place and a vital place it is." He mentioned the pension systems of some of the more progressive business concerns, but said that it was now necessary for government "to take a hand." He indicated that the Administration's program did increase public attention to the problem (this seems to reverse cause and effect) but that it was "complicated legislation the Administration rushed through in characteristic fashion." [35]

The reluctance of political parties officially to criticize the principle of government intervention did not prevent a bitter tone from entering into the official criticism of the Social Security Act. The keynote speech to the Republican convention included attacks upon every major New Deal measure except stock market legislation and social security,[36] and it was not long before those who attacked the New Deal began to attack the Act as well.

THE REACTION

The first concerted attack upon the social security program took the form of notices included by many employers with the pay envelopes of their employees. During the campaign of 1936, workers throughout the country found slips with their pay charging that the new program was merely a method of increasing tax revenues. These notices typically failed even to mention the benefits due the employee, or that the employer was to pay one-half of the tax for Old-Age Insurance. Joseph P. Kennedy, then Chairman of the Securities and Exchange Commission, charged that the pay-envelope campaign was grossly unfair and false, and that it attempted to "create the impression that giving old age insurance at half-price to the worker is an unfair tax on the worker." [37] The President, in an address at Madison Square Garden on October 31, attacked the employers engaging in the pay-envelope effort for deceit in neglecting to tell the complete story, and for attempting to coerce their workers into voting against him.[38] He said that two "policies" were provided by the Act, unemployment insurance to be paid for by the employer, and the old age program paid for jointly by the employer and the employee. On the second of November, the New York Herald Tribune called Roosevelt's speech "bitter and defiant." In Middletown, the Lynds found that "Landon and higher wages" was the basis of the attack.[39] The factories there distributed notices with their pay checks emphasizing the deductions from pay that would result from the Social Security Act. The envelope-stuffers charged that the scheme would make pay raises impossible, and that the system, in all likelihood, would soon collapse. They did not mention the benefits to the workers.

Some of the most bitter criticism of Roosevelt and the New Deal came from the Hearst newspapers. An example is an editorial that appeared in late May discussing Landon's views on social security:

> He is careful to imply that it . . . must be along AMERICAN lines, and not to be a detail in a general scheme such as this Administration has put forth, to reduce millions of Americans to the condition of STATE PARASITES. In fact, one great fault of Mr. Roosevelt is that he has, by his extreme and extravagant methods, discredited all progressive ideas. Governor Landon, however, indicates that no social security legislation based on COLLECTIVIST DELUSIONS or that is plainly UNCONSTITUTIONAL will receive his assent.[40]

Attacks such as this forced the President, in a speech at Syracuse in September 1936, to defend the Social Security Act against charges of being "radical and alien." [41] At the same time, Governor Landon was working hard to bring his own state under the protection of all portions of the Act; he called a special session of the Kansas Legislature for July 7, 1936 to begin work upon a constitutional amendment allowing Kansas to participate.

The most severe criticisms came not from political parties but from groups with special interests. The statement issued by Henry Ford in 1936 was typical of much of this criticism:

> Under some social security systems abroad a man cannot quit his job, or apply for another, or leave town and go to another even to get a better job because that would break the 'economic plan.' Such a restriction of liberty will be almost a necessity in this country too if the present Social Security Act works to its natural conclusions.[42]

At that time, the United States Chamber of Commerce took a somewhat more moderate viewpoint, and expressed it in a "Statement of Principles" said to represent the opinions of its

1,400 member organizations including some 700,000 members. Of social security, the Chamber said:

> Business would ignore its gravest responsibility if it failed to provide the greatest possible degree of economic security to the individual. The attainment of this end so necessary to the furtherance of American ideals will require not only the maintenance of high wages but likewise a constructive solution to the complex problem of security to the individual when he or she has outlived capacity to earn a comfortable living. Here again interference by government in attempts to reduce the whole complex problem to one of legislative formulae can only postpone the final solution by making it more difficult for business to assume its own obligations in the matter.[43]

The remarks of Professor Raymond Pearl of John Hopkins University, then president of the American Statistical Association, illustrate the extreme nature of some of the criticism. In December, 1939, Dr. Pearl—who was himself sixty years of age at the time—suggested that, by their advocacy of old age pension "nostrums," the aged may be proving themselves too foolish to be allowed the privilege of voting. He said that the aged together with the young "are ganging up on the half of the population that does the work." He said that the demands of the young had decreased somewhat, but that the increase in the proportion of persons who have "finished whatever biological justification there ever was for existence" constituted a social problem of the first magnitude.[44]

Several critics spoke well of the purposes of the Act, while criticizing its provisions. The editors of *Collier's* said that "few have quarreled with the broad purposes underlying the Social Security Act. On the other hand, many of the most experienced and sincere advocates of social insurance are aghast at some of the provisions. . . ."[45] Winthrop W. Aldrich, then chairman of the board of directors of the Chase National Bank, echoed these sentiments saying that many were sympathetic to the objectives of the Act, but that its form created a "grave menace to the future security of the country as a whole and to the security of the very people it is designed to protect." [46]

Writers today often mention the opposition of "extremist" groups, such as the charges by the Liberty League that the system was unworkable, and have seemingly forgotten that the same charge was a part of the 1936 Republican platform.[47] Again, this was opposition specifically to the Social Security Act, and not necessarily to the basic principles of social insurance. It seems clear, however, that the social security programs and the public support for the Social Security Act definitely contributed a major impetus to the repudiation of the Republicans in 1936. Although many prominent Republicans favored the Act or advocated similar programs, and the party officially had taken a position less extreme than that taken by many industrial leaders, the mood of the public called for more action than the Republicans could offer. The final vote in the House was 372 in favor of the Act (288 Democrats, 77 Republicans, 6 Progressives, and 1 Farmer-Labor), and 33 opposed (13 Democrats, 18 Republicans, and 2 Farmer-Labor). In the Senate the final vote was 77 in favor (60 Democrats, 15 Republicans, 1 Progressive, and 1 Farmer-Labor), and 6 (1 Democrat and 5 Republicans) opposed; but the Republicans just prior to this voted 12 to 8 to eliminate Old-Age Insurance.[48]

PUBLIC OPINION

There are still individual criticisms of the social security programs by political figures, especially when Congress considers adding benefits, but neither party has criticized the Act officially since 1936. Most observers believe that this would be politically perilous, since the American public now seems to accept social security as a part of the "American way of life." In his noted work on public opinion, V. O. Key, Jr. says that the acceptance of the basic social security principles renders attacks upon the system profitless, making the "burning issues . . . much narrower than the existence of the program." [49] Since

1950, every election year except 1964 has seen significant legislation expanding coverage or adding benefits. In 1964, both houses passed a bill extending the system, but it was lost when the conference committee failed to agree regarding a health-care amendment adopted by the Senate. Though not infallible, the major political parties generally may be assumed to have judged accurately the wishes of the people when they repeatedly cooperate to extend a program—especially during election years.

It seems indisputable that Americans generally have favored the programs of the Social Security Act since its adoption. This is indicated not only by the behavior of the political parties, but by the public acceptance of steadily increasing tax rates; it is also the unanimous opinion of the experts on social insurance. Certain factors not necessarily central to the principles of social insurance favor this acceptance. For instance, the Old Age, Survivors', and Disability Insurance portions of the program are financed through trust funds and do not directly affect the "balancing" of the federal budget, as it is ordinarily measured.

Ironically, in view of their usual opposition to the program, the insurance companies have probably contributed considerably to the acceptance of social security (OASDI) by adopting sales techniques that center upon social security as the base upon which to build private insurance protection. A brief session with a life insurance salesman often teaches a prospective customer the value of this social security coverage, and as a by-product gives him some indication of the expense that would be involved if he were to duplicate it privately.

One set of material typical of insurance company advertising contained a form letter, headed by a drawing of a social security account number card beneath block lettering asking, "HOW MUCH MONEY DO YOU HAVE COMING TO YOU UNDER THE *NEW* SOCIAL SECURITY BENEFITS?" Followed by, "Send for FREE Benefit-Selector Guide from Mutual of Omaha!" The text stressed the avoidance of possible loss by getting the "latest facts" from the insurance company. The company offered to send not only the "details of a low-cost Plan for . . . security and peace of mind" but a "newly revised Social Security Benefit-Selector Guide" for "fast, easy reference." It assured that the company merely wished the recipient to have on hand the "details of this modern way to protect" his income. The Guide could be used to "spin out" the answers to such questions as:

1. What are the new Social Security Benefits for men?
2. What are the new Benefits for women?
3. Am I eligible for the new Benefits?
4. How much will I receive if I become disabled?
5. What must I do to avoid losing any Benefits?

This is an excellent example of the publicity given social security by the promotional activities of the insurance companies.

The corporate pension plans that are based upon the principles of adding to a base of social security payments have also, in all likelihood, helped to publicize the program favorably. Moreover, the Social Security Administration itself conducts impressive publicity programs. Though these efforts ostensibly are directed toward informing the people of their rights under the programs, and not toward building up favorable responses, they inevitably have this result also. The informational activities range from those of the field representatives in the more than six hundred district offices to the sponsorship of "The World of Folk Music," a series of radio broadcasts featuring specially recorded songs by well-known folk singers and including general discussions of social security.

The public opinion polls beginning with that by Dr. Gallup's American Institute of Public Opinion (AIPO) in December 1935, further reinforce the contention that social security programs have been very well received. Virtually every major poll dealing with the principles of social security during the program's existence has indicated strong public support.[50] This reflects a sharp change in opinion. "Prior to the great depression," says Paul Douglas, "the consensus of public opinion [*sic*] was that American citizens could in the main provide for their old age by individual savings." [51]

In a series of AIPO polls taken from December 1935 to November 1939, no less than 89 per cent of those interviewed said that they were in favor of "government old age pensions for needy persons." The question asked in July 1941 deleted the phrase "for needy persons." As before, the vast majority of those polled (91 per cent) professed their support.[52]

The results of the polls also reinforce the belief that the support of the Act was essentially bi-partisan. In the poll of December 1935, 94.5 per cent of the Democrats and 80 per cent of the Republicans favored pensions, though the question limited the subject to needy persons.[53] Leaving the general for the specific, the interviewers asked, "Do you favor the compulsory old age insurance plan, starting January 1, which requires employers and employees to make equal monthly contributions?" The responses in September and November 1936 and January 1937 were respectively 68 percent, 69 per cent, and 77 per cent in favor.[54]

In January 1947, Elmo Roper conducted a poll similar to those conducted by Gallup's AIPO to test the most- and least-liked features of the Roosevelt Administration.[55] His results were similar to those of Dr. Gallup. In Roper's poll, 15 per cent listed social security legislation as the most-liked features of the New Deal, as compared with Gallup's 14 per cent, but whereas on the AIPO poll it had been named more often than any other single subject, several ranked ahead of it on the poll by Roper. Both improvement of the labor situation (16 per cent) and banking and investment controls (19 per cent) led social security. Topping the list, however, was "interest in the welfare of the common man" (28 per cent). This category is sufficiently imprecise to include any social welfare measure, and might have been named by some who would otherwise have listed Social Security. At any rate, social security ranked high on both lists of well-liked measures, and did not appear on either list of those that were not approved. This was consistent with Roper's findings in 1945 that 77 per cent of those polled thought that it would be a good idea to extend Social Security to everyone who had a job.[56]

THE SOCIAL SECURITY ACT TODAY

The programs under the Social Security Act have broadened throughout the years. The act now includes Old Age, Survivors', and Disability Insurance (Title II), Grants to States for Old Age Assistance and Medical Assistance for the Aged (Title I), Grants to States for Unemployment Compensation Administration (Title III), Grants to States for Aid and Services to needy Families with Children (Title IV), Grants to States for Maternal and Child Welfare (Title V), Grants to States for Aid to the Blind (Title X), Grants to States for Aid to the Permanently and Totally Disabled (Title XIV), Grants to States for Aid to the Aged, Blind or Disabled, or for Such Aid and Medical Assistance for the Aged (Title XVI—the "Kerr-Mills Act"), the Medicare provisions (Title XVIII), as well as other, more limited, programs. The only major programs administered entirely by the federal government are those of contributory social insurance, as was true in 1935. With this major exception, the original act was, and the present act is, almost completely one of grants-in-aid to the states.

The original contributory insurance program was established to achieve the benefits of a social insurance system through a mechanism built primarily, though certainly not exclusively, upon a contractual-fiscal basis. The major criticisms at its establishment verify this. The critics pointed out that it delayed benefits for years after taxes began, that its benefits were very low, that it covered too few risks and too few persons, and that the reserves contemplated were unnecessary and so high as to be dangerous.[57] The emphasis upon the contractual nature of social security, incidentally, is so patently inapplicable under current judicial interpretation that present supporters of the system attempt to avoid it.[58] The changes in the act have not entirely eliminated the older principles upon which the program was established, but there have been changes in orientation. Even though these changes are readily evident from an examination of the provisions of the system and their changing character, the image of the program, and the terms used to describe it, have not varied at all from those at its beginning.

It seems indisputable that the Social Security Act of 1935 represented an innovation in American political action. It is true that its programs, including contributory social insurance, were far from perfect. It is impossible to refute the charge, for example, that the insurance-company model forces the poor (elderly or otherwise) "to pay most of the cost of keeping the poor." [59] But regardless of its faults, the act did at least represent a belated acknowledgment of something beyond "civil" and "political" rights; it gave legal sanction to the notion that every person has definite social rights.[60]

THE MISSING BENEFIT

In the three decades between the passage of the Social Security Act and the incorporation of "Medicare," many students of social insurance and related subjects pointed to the absence of provisions for health care as the most notable weakness of the social security system in the United States. Beginning shortly after its passage, a series of attempts ensued to broaden the act to include some form of health care, or to establish independent health care programs aided in varying degrees by the federal government. Opposition of American "organized medicine"—most notably the American Medical Association and its affiliates, and a number of state and regional organizations of medical practitioners—to federal "interference" in matters of individual and public health began long before 1935 and cannot be attributed to fear that the Social Security Act in particular might become a vehicle for "government medicine." But the Social Security Act and related legislation did intensify fears that already existed, and gave rise to increased efforts by medical organizations to challenge and defeat any and all laws that might call into question the physician's traditional position in American society as the sole and unquestioned authority on all matters pertaining to health and medical care.

In retrospect it is hard to see how inclusion of health benefits in the original Social Security Act could have represented a more "radical" departure from American tradition than did its unemployment and old age benefits. Nevertheless, two factors prevented this inclusion. The first was the obvious preoccupation with the question of monetary income and specifically the fact that for most people such income ceased to come in after retirement. The second was the traditional viewpoint of organized medicine. The President's Committee on Economic Security studied the health care issue at length, but mentioned it only briefly in its report. At no time did the Social Security Bill include any item relating to health insurance except one calling for further study.[61]

According to Professor Edwin Witte, Executive Director of the Committee on Economic Security, leaders of organized medicine were suspicious that the Administration was attempting to use the committee to bring about the passage of governmental health insurance. The original assignment of duties to the committee had included the responsibility to study the question of health insurance as a portion of the overall question of economic security. The Administration did not press the issue because, according to Secretary of Labor Frances Perkins, the opposition from the American Medical Association was so great that any inclusion of health-care provisions could have prevented passage of the entire Social Security Bill.[62]

In August 1934, when it first became known that the committee's research would include a study of governmental health insurance, the President received numerous telegrams protesting such a study. These telegrams and criticism in the medical journals prompted him to appoint a Medical Advisory Committee including the presidents of the American Medical Association and the American College of Surgeons, and the vice-president of the American College of Physicians. (The president was a Canadian.) Other professional organizations, such as the American Osteopathic Association and the National Medical Association, a group of Negro physicians, were not represented on the Committee. Nor were the homeopaths and chiropractors. These omissions gave rise to vigorous protests on the part of the unrepresented groups but in the judgment of Professor Witte including them would have further alienated the "major" medical organizations.[63]

Before the end of the day on which the appointments to the group were announced (November 4, 1934), the President received hundreds of telegrams protesting that he had included neither a general practitioner nor a physician from the Rocky Mountain area. All those complaining of the lack of a physician from the Rocky Mountain area suggested a Denver physician who had been an outspoken critic of health insurance. Witte says that the telegrams generally came in batches from certain sections of the country and that many of them were identical in wording. He mentions also that medical journals throughout the nation published critical editorials.[64]

An incident that occurred at a "round table on medical care" at the Secretary of Labor's National Conference on Economic Security, that began in Washington on November 14, 1934, illustrates both the attitude of much of organized medicine and the tactics to which it frequently has resorted. The four physicians on the round table had been selected so that a balance would result between proponents and opponents of health insurance, but one of the two who had been scheduled to speak in favor of a governmental health program instead spoke very critically. Dr. James D. Bruce, a member of the Medical Advisory Committee, the next day charged that the American Medical Association had been responsible for this abrupt change of opinion. He presented evidence that indicated that the speaker, a physician from Detroit, had been subject to a professional boycott (that is, other physicians were refusing to refer patients to him or to consult with him) since his attitude had become known to the Michigan State Medical Association, and that a representative from the Chicago office of the American Medical Association had called upon him and informed him that the boycott might end if he were to attack governmental health care in his talk at the National Conference. Several members of the Medical Advisory Committee then informed Dr. Walter L. Bierring, the president of the American Medical Association, that the association was in danger of being "split wide open" if its tactics did not change. Dr. Bierring gave assurances that the association would work with the Medical Advisory Committee, and thereafter, for a time, a truce existed.[65]

Dr. Morris Fishbein, editor of the *Journal of the American Medical Association,* and one of the association's most vociferous and articulate critics of all changes in the organization of medical services, published an editorial expressing confidence in the Committee on Economic Security and the Medical Advisory Committee. Witte remarks that the optimism which the truce aroused in the Committee on Economic Security seems to have arisen from a misinterpretation of the attitude of the Medical Advisory Committee, which was more to heal a split in the profession than to endorse a governmental health program.[66] This split in the profession was a severe one. In addition to the fight against governmental involvement, there was an internal struggle involving group practice, health insurance, and the varied interests of specialists as opposed to general practitioners.

The report of the President's Committee on Economic Security (published on January 15, 1935) was alleged by many medical journals to be an endorsement of government health insurance, and many physicians apparently gained the impression that the ensuing bill, the Economic Security Bill, included provisions relating to health care. The American Medical Association thereupon called a special meeting of its House of Delegates—the first such meeting since World War I—for consideration of the question of health insurance and specifically the recommendations of the President's Committee. According to Witte, this special session did much to create something close to unanimity among the association's members. For the first time, the association went on record as endorsing experimentation with voluntary health plans to be supervised and controlled by local and state medical societies. At the same time, it reaffirmed its opposition to any form of "compulsory" health insurance and to "lay control" of medical services. This action served to unite most of the membership in opposition to legislation providing for establishment of a federal health program. Consequently, groups that formerly had been more or less inclined to support some such program immediately withdrew their support—ostensibly so that the association's recommendations could receive a fair trial. The American College of Surgeons, for example, in 1934 had strongly endorsed governmental health insurance (at least in principle), but at its convention in 1935 the organization ignored the subject completely.

Such indications that the medical profession was becoming more united in its opposition to a government health care program aroused considerable anxiety among the members of the House Ways and Means Committee, which was then considering the Economic Security Bill. The opposition of organized medicine, in fact, seems to have been a major factor in the omission of health benefits, or any mention of them, from the Social Security Act of 1935.

At the first executive session of the Ways and Means Committee following the special meeting of the American Medical Association's House of Delegates mentioned above, the committee members asked that sections of the bill providing for health benefits be pointed out to them. They were told that the bill contained no such provisions. The only mention of health care was found in a clause dealing with the responsibilities of the Social Security Board; in addition to administering the Social Security program, if such were brought into being, the proposed board was to study possible future extensions of Social Security, including the possible addition of some kind of health insurance program. Forthwith, the committee voted unanimously to delete the offensive passage, eliminating all that might be construed as having to do with health benefits. However, as Witte notes, many congressmen continued to receive letters of protest from physicians who were still under the impression that the Economic Security Bill provided for some kind of health insurance—when, in point of fact, it had *never* done anything of the kind.

Though the Committee on Economic Security had recommended the creation of a governmental health benefits program in a report sent to the President on November 6, 1934, this report and its recommendation were never publicized and health insurance was not incorporated into the bill. Sometime later, after forming the Social Security Board, the President sent the report to the membership suggesting that they might wish to be informed on the subject.[67]

For years, any suggestion of a change in the government's attitude toward medical care had called forth extreme and immediate reactions from the American Medical Association. As early (or as late) as 1932, for example, Dr. Morris Fishbein was charging that medical care provided by organized medical groups (that is, "group practice," as recommended by the Committee on the Costs of Medical Care) represented "medical soviets." [68]

In 1940, the association's president elect, Nathan B. Van Etten, sounded the alarm. If "paganism" won out in Europe, he declared, the United States would be required to resist it strongly—and "the subversive influence of so-called 'fifth columns,' *already here*" would "grow stronger *in our national administration . . .*" [emphasis supplied]. Oliver Garceau, a political scientist then at Harvard, points out the thinly veiled criticism of reformism as being alien and subversive. He concludes that the association revised its tactics to suit the wartime era; to use its wartime functions to close the gaps in its ranks and to attack its opponents.[69]

In response to President Truman's health-care message of 1949, the AMA released a statement saying that there was no hope of progress in "this system of regimented medical care" and that it was the "discredited system of decadent nations which are now living off the bounty of the American people— and if adopted it would not only jeopardize the health of our people but would gravely endanger our freedom. It is one of the final, irrevocable steps toward state socialism—and every American should be alerted to the danger." [70]

In December 1951, the AMA's House of Delegates called for an investigation of the nation's "entire school system" to expose teachers and authors of textbooks that would undermine free enterprise by upholding the "fallacies of collectivism." Moreover, it called for the removal of any teacher or textbook deemed to support "collectivistic thought," presumably leaving the determination and the definition to the investigator.[71] Time and again the American Medical Association has charged the physicians of the country to make use of their prestige and their image as persons of authority to preach moral regeneration through political and economic conservatism, as the terms are popularly understood, especially, but certainly not exclusively, in matters of governmental involvement in the supplying of health services to the general population.

To this end there has been at least an informal alliance between the American Medical Association and the United States Chamber of Commerce to combat specifically the extension of social security to cover health benefits, and by implication to criticize the social security programs, other governmental activities, and to further the political ideals of the two organizations. The Chamber and the association have each distributed the other's literature on the health-care subject, and the association's House of Delegates adopted a resolution in

1961 recommending that state and local medical societies support chambers of commerce at all levels in "promoting the free-enterprise system." [72]

Physicians are extremely busy men and often have little time for intellectual inquiry beyond the confines of their practice. They, therefore, are inclined to look to their professional organization for guidance, and the association has never been reluctant to supply it. Oliver Garceau, in fact, went so far as to say, in 1940, that the services provided by the American Medical Association were well calculated to save the physician the "awkward predicament of having to think." [73] Though this may be stated immoderately, Garceau points out that the physician had available to him an association clipping bureau and package service, assistance in supplying the outlines of lectures and radio addresses, and pamphlets giving the association's views upon controversial issues. This kind of assistance has been greatly increased with the growth of the health-care question as a political issue. John Detar, a Michigan physician, wrote a pamphlet, "The Country Doctor Answers the Ewing Report," that is only one of many typical examples. This document, published in 1950 by the Michigan Medical Society, contains an index-like code that tells the physician which paragraphs to paste together as the basis for any talk, depending upon the length of the talk and the character of the audience. [74]

As a counterpart to such assistance for the physician, the American Medical Association has attempted to shield him from any controversy within its own ranks that would call into question any of its official positions. Though the *Journal of the American Medical Association (JAMA)* did print an article by then-Senator Hubert Humphrey endorsing the Kennedy Administration's Anderson-King plan, it has consistently refused to take note of the existence of the small group of physicians also supporting the idea of governmental health insurance. In printing the article by Mr. Humphrey, a well-known advocate of Medicare, the Association ran little danger of introducing dissent within its own ranks, especially in light of the classic disregard of the physician for the opinion of a "layman" in matters remotely relating to health care.

To carry material favorable to the plan if written by a layman is one thing; if written by a physician, it is quite another. In May 1962, a physician, Dr. Caldwell B. Esselstyn, chairman of a group of physicians supporting the Anderson-King Bill, criticized the Association severely for refusing to carry an advertisement by his group in either the *JAMA* or the *AMA News*. He told a news conference that the refusal was inconsistent with the Association's slogan of "free choice" and said, "This stand is consistent with the policy of protecting the AMA members from any exposure to an unemotional presentation of facts proving the necessity and the need for financing certain basic costs of the aged through social security." [75]

Perhaps this general orientation is a partial explanation for the stream of letters from physicians and dentists to any magazine printing material questioning organized medicine's basic assumptions, letters that often fail to confine themselves to a discussion of the issues, and cancel or threaten to cancel subscriptions. When a physician, David Rutstein, had the temerity to question the foundations of the Association-supported Kerr-Mills program in an article entitled "The Medical Care Pork Barrel" in the *Atlantic Monthly,* that magazine received the usual letters from physicians questioning the wisdom of continuing their subscriptions. One letter, typical of many resulting whenever policies of the American Medical Association are criticized, illustrates the social and political role that many physicians see for themselves, and that the Association explicitly propagates. This letter charged Dr. Rutstein with having lost sight of the "purposes of organization" of the United States, and with being either "content to work on salary" or "too timid to practice independent medicine." It proceeds to say that we have been so "infiltrated and propagandized by those who insist that we must become part of the herd" that the last truly independent segment of our society, the "last bastion of individualism, the medical profession," is endangered.[76]

Throughout their formal propaganda campaigns, as earlier during the 1930's, the Association has relied heavily upon the use of slogans and epithets calculated to encourage emotionalism and discourage thought. It has used the term "socialism," virtually a political swear-word in the United States, to maximum advantage. A popular slogan of the National Education Campaign was "Guard your health—Guard your pocketbook—Socialized Medicine would rob both." Then, as now, a favorite allusion was to governmental health insurance as the "entering wedge" for socialized medicine, or the latest illustration of the prevalence of "creeping socialism." Since that time, the AMA has characterized as socialistic even such mild measures as federal re-insurance of voluntary health insurance plans and permanent and total disability insurance under social security (though it is to the association's credit that since the latter has been adopted it has cooperated fully with the Social Security Administration regarding the program). A visual manifestation of the verbal tendency to arouse emotion rather than thought was the Association's distribution of Sir Luke Fildes' painting "The Doctor" with the admonition to "keep politics out of this picture." As evidence of the soundness of the tactical judgments underlying organized medicine's campaigns, it may be noted that they remained markedly successful for years.

IV

the struggle for medicare

As mentioned earlier, from 1915 to 1918 organized medicine seemed to receive calmly some suggestions that a program of governmental health benefits might be advantageous for the United States; the subcommittee on social insurance of the American Medical Association's Council on Health and Public Instruction even issued some favorable reports. By the end of 1919, however, there was a concerted attack upon the Council and upon I. M. Rubinow, the secretary of the social insurance subcommittee. The "official history" of the association by Morris Fishbein reports that "many of the statements presented in the pamphlets published by the Council could be found in the propaganda issued by the American Association for Labor Legislation," and that the American Medical Association "discovered" that Dr. Rubinow was simultaneously in the employ of that pro-social-insurance group.[1] In 1920, at the annual House of Delegates meeting held that year in New Orleans, after a vigorous attack upon the association's president, Alexander Lambert (who was also a member of both the social insurance subcommittee and the American Association for Labor Legislation),[2] the association formally adopted the following resolution:

> *Resolved,* That the American Medical Association declares its opposition to the institution of any plan embodying the system

of compulsory contributory insurance against illness, or any other
plan of compulsory insurance which provides for medical service
to be rendered contributors or their dependents, provided, controlled or regulated by any state or the federal government.

Fishbein's official history, published in 1947, declared that this
had remained the policy of the association since 1920.[3]

Though the association's policy of strenuous opposition began
as early as 1920, the issue lay dormant until the Committee on
the Costs of Medical Care released its majority report in 1932.
The efforts of supporters of governmental health insurance during the New Deal period brought the subject to serious political
discussion. Since then, it has repeatedly emerged as a major
political issue.[4]

In 1939, Senator Wagner of New York introduced a proposal
to establish a national health program providing grants to the
states, which were to develop health plans conforming to federal
standards. Similar bills had been introduced previously but this
was the first to receive serious consideration. The subcommittee
examining the bill issued a favorable interim report, the American Medical Association produced twenty-two arguments
against it, and there was no further action.[5]

In 1943, the first of a series of Wagner-Murray-Dingell Bills
was proposed. This bill would have established a national system of hospitals and medical benefits, financed by a payroll tax
on employers and employees. It would have provided the patient
with free choice of participating physicians and authorized the
Surgeon General of the Public Health Service to set fee sched-
ules and regulate the number of patients each physician would
treat. The reaction from organized medicine was immediate and
hostile. The National Physicians Committee charged that "the
processes proposed and the mechanisms indicated are designed
to act as the catalyst in transforming a rapidly expanding Federal bureaucracy into an all powerful totalitarian state control.
Human rights as opposed to slavery is the issue." [6] The bill
never emerged from committee. A similar fate lay in store for
the next Wagner-Murray-Dingell Bill in 1945, even though it

had strong support from the Truman Administration. The Republican Eightieth Congress considered a revised Wagner-Murray-Dingell Bill in 1947. Both this and the 1945 version provided for state administration of a federal program.

The last major Truman Administration health bill was that of 1949. This bill, similar to the Wagner-Murray-Dingell Bill of 1947, was based upon the Federal Security Agency's report to the President, *The Nation's Health, A Ten-Year Program,* by Oscar Ewing. During the campaign of 1948, the President had strongly urged the adoption of the principles of the Ewing Report, and the election returns heightened the anxiety of many members of the American Medical Association.

As alternatives to the programs of the Administration, Senator Robert A. Taft (R-Ohio) sponsored a series of bills in 1946, 1947, and 1949 calling for state-operated programs of aid to those unable to pay for health care. The provisions of these bills were similar to those of the Kerr-Mills Act ("Medical Aid to the Aged"), except that they were not limited to the elderly. The American Medical Association did not attack the Taft bills, but failed to support them because of displeasure at the prospect of lay administration at the local level.[7]

The attitude of opposition by the American Medical Association had begun as far back as 1920, and with the renewal of the issue in the 1930's, the association's pronouncements came to be characterized by extreme language frequently linking any suggestion not to the liking of organized medicine to socialism and communism and even specifically to the Soviet Union. The continuous, unified, massive campaign, however, arose during the 1940's, as did organized medicine's strategic pattern of opposition. Before this time, the opposition had taken varying forms, apparently as disconnected responses to events rather than as a concerted effort to halt a general tendency toward a governmental program.

From 1939 to 1948, the American Medical Association expressed its opposition through the National Physicians Committee for the Extension of Medical Service (NPC), which had come into existence in response to the Wagner Bill of 1939. The American Medical Association denied any connection with NPC, but AMA members headed it, and AMA fund-raising mechanisms supported it. Both the profession and the public considered the NPC to be the AMA spokesman, and presumably it was formed because of fears that the AMA's charter as a non-profit organization would prevent it from lobbying extensively. (In view of the extent of direct lobbying by the AMA in recent years, it seems safe to assume that its fears on this account have been, at least partially, laid to rest.) During the NPC's existence, the AMA confined its official activities of opposition to speeches, editorials, legislative testimony, and resolutions by its House of Delegates.

The NPC worked through physicians' offices to distribute a huge number of pamphlets and other printed material concerning governmental health insurance. By 1948, however, its influence had waned, owing to a growing reaction against some of its propaganda tactics and public distaste for "radical right" groups with which it had associated itself.[8]

In 1946 the AMA decided to hire a special public relations counsel, thus taking its first official step toward cleansing its reputation. And in 1949 Dr. Fishbein, who had been intimately involved in the association's opposition to health insurance, and specifically with much of the extreme language used by the Association since the early 1930's, retired as editor of *JAMA* after considerable criticism from within the profession that he had been responsible for a great deal of the tarnish on the professional image.

As indicated earlier, organized medicine had reacted with alarm to the Truman victory of 1948. It therefore began extensive efforts to launch strong and positive programs of opposition to governmental health insurance and to appeal to the citizenry for support. With great haste the House of Delegates levied an assessment of twenty-five dollars on each member to build a three and one-half million dollar "political war chest to fight socialized medicine." It planned a "National Education

Campaign" (advertising) to "educate" the American people and hired the public relations firm of Whitaker and Baxter to direct it. The National Education Campaign successfully overcame opposition within the association to the assessment, and virtually all members displayed posters and distributed pamphlets to patients. Physicians and their wives (the latter were instructed to "tuck pamphlets into all . . . personal correspondence—even invitations to dinner parties"—but to avoid debates) distributed some twenty million pamphlets in the first year. Additionally, the personal physicians of members of Congress urged them to support AMA views. Cooperating with the physicians were (among others) insurance agents and companies, dentists, and pharmacists.

The 1949 campaign, according to Whitaker and Baxter, resulted in the distribution of fifty-five million pieces of literature reaching approximately one hundred million persons. Coupled with the attacks upon governmental programs was a successful emphasis on promotion of commercial health insurance policies under the slogan "The Voluntary Way is the American Way." [9] The techniques were new, skillful, and thorough. The major arguments in this and subsequent campaigns differed little, however, from those that Morris Fishbein used extensively and elaborated fully during the 1930's; they arose from medicine, not Madison Avenue.

The 1950 campaign made use of the same techniques that had proved to be so effective in 1949. In addition, physicians formed political committees in many congressional districts. In Wisconsin, for example, "Physicians for Freedom" helped defeat Andrew Biemiller (D-Wisc.), in his campaign for re-election to the House of Representatives by using posters, advertisements, and campaign literature included with monthly bills to patients. Biemiller was an outspoken proponent of health care legislation. Similarly, Senator Claude Pepper (D-Fla.) lost his campaign for re-election partly as a result of organized medicine's opposition, which gave rise to such tactics as those practiced by the Tallahassee hospital that placed cards reading "This is the season for canning Pepper" on patients' breakfast trays.[10]

In 1952, an organization calling itself the "National Professional Committee for Eisenhower and Nixon" mailed its political literature from the address of the former National Education Campaign. Though the AMA was officially neutral in the election, the National Professional Committee used letterheads listing former AMA president Elmer L. Henderson as chairman and former presidents John Wesley Cline and Ernest F. Irons as vice-chairmen, and also included the names of Whitaker and Baxter. A similar "Physicians for Stevenson" organization had no AMA officials as sponsors, or any other evidence of AMA support.[11] With the election of a Republican administration avowedly hostile to governmental health insurance, which it agreed was "socialized medicine," the formal public relations or propaganda campaigns financed by the AMA lessened in intensity.

The AMA was placed on the alert again in 1957 by the introduction of the first Forand Bill (H.R. 9467). This was a proposal by Representative Aime Forand (D-R.I.) to pay for certain hospital and surgical services that were rendered to persons receiving social security benefits. Forand re-introduced his bill into the 86th Congress in 1959 (H.R. 4700). The House Ways and Means Committee held hearings on Forand's bills in 1957, 1958, and 1959 but took no action. On March 31, 1960, the Committee finally rejected the plan by a vote of seventeen to eight—ironically, the same vote by which it was to accept the Medicare proposal five years later. In the same year, Senator John F. Kennedy (D-Mass.) introduced a bill similar to those introduced by Representative Forand, and after his nomination for the presidency, made his support of the measure a major campaign point. His bill failed in the Senate by a vote of fifty-five to forty-one, defeated by a coalition of Republicans and southern Democrats. In 1961, the Ways and Means Committee again held hearings—and again took no action.

AMA opposition to Medicare during the Kennedy Administration reached a peak in 1962 in response to the Anderson-King Bill, sponsored by Representative Cecil King (D-Calif.) and Senator Clinton Anderson (D-N.M.). This campaign and the subsequent efforts of opponents of government health insurance are discussed in detail in the next chapter.

The Anderson-King Bill would have provided direct payment to hospitals for services rendered to social security beneficiaries aged sixty-five and over. Such services were to be limited to the costs of up to ninety days (per "benefit period") of care in hospitals that had signed agreements with the government. The beneficiary was to pay from twenty to ninety dollars, depending upon the length of his stay. The bill also would have provided payment for certain nursing home, home health, and outpatient diagnostic services, but it did not include payment for physicians' services except those customarily considered part of hospital care. The beneficiary's choice of physician would have been unaffected, as would the choice of hospital (assuming that the patient's physician had staff privileges at a hospital that had agreed to accept payment from the program). The benefits were to have been financed by an increase of one fourth of one per cent in the social security tax on employers and employees. The bill was designed to avoid any changes in the organization of medical and hospital practice.

The provisions of the Anderson-King Bill were modified in the second session of the Eighty-seventh Congress, and supporters attempted to attach the revised measure, as the Anderson-Javits amendment, to a House-approved public-welfare bill. Opponents defeated the attempt by tabling the amendment in July 1962. This was the climax of the controversy over Medicare, before its passage by the Eighty-ninth Congress.

In September 1964, the Senate adopted an amendment to the Social Security Act similar to the Anderson-Javits amendment, as detailed later; but its destiny was death in the conference committee. This was not accompanied by the intensive public campaign that surrounded the Anderson-King and Anderson-Javits proposals, probably because the opponents were sure of themselves. The only other favorable action on even a slightly related health care program before the Eighty-ninth Congress came in 1960 when Congress adopted the Kerr-Mills Act (actually an amendment to the Social Security Act, becoming Title XVI "Medical Aid to the Aged") providing grants to the states to assist in the health needs of the indigent and the "medically indigent" aged. The AMA supported this as a means of averting action upon the Forand bill, or some other program of broader scope.

This support was the first sign of a crack in the solid front presented by organized medicine against any extension of governmental involvement in either health care or its economics. The crack was very small, but it ultimately widened to include an intensive AMA effort in support of its own "eldercare" program, which also called for federal support. Further evidence was not long in coming, and resulted from actions taken by hospitals and their representative groups rather than by organized medicine. During the most fierce of the Medicare campaigns, the president of the Blue Cross Association, Walter J. McNerney, announced a Blue Cross proposal that he called "without a doubt more liberal and inclusive" than that suggested by the Administration. It would have provided uniform benefits at uniform rates to all persons aged sixty-five and over, with subsidies from the government to assist those who needed them to pay the premiums. This plan would have provided only seventy days of hospitalization as opposed to the Administration bill's ninety, and it would not have incorporated the payment of a deductible. The estimated cost was ten to twelve dollars per month per person. The basic details of the plan (as announced January 3, 1962) had been worked out by Blue Cross in cooperation with the American Hospital Association. On January 4, the AHA's House of Delegates announced its support for the measure, "conditional upon the administration of the

proposed plan by the voluntary non-profit pre-payment system"
—that is, by the Blue Cross groups. The statement added that
the source of funds was of "secondary importance." With this
phrase, the major American hospital organization had, for the
first time, broken officially with the AMA on the crucial question
of the financing of health care.

The AMA's response indicated no change in its attitude.
The association said that it was interested to learn that the
hospital group had "gone on record that the best interests of
the aged would not be served by the King-Anderson bill, and
the House of Delegates opposed the use of the social security
mechanism for the administration of any form of health care
for the aged."

On January 17, the AMA announced a plan of its own: a
national insurance program for the elderly under the auspices
of the Blue Shield plans. This would provide for payment of
the physicians' bills at a uniform cost to the beneficiary of
three dollars per month. The executive vice-president of the
Blue Shield organization, John W. Castellucci, said that he
hoped that the plan could be advertised as early as April and
be put in effect by July. First, however, it had to be approved
by the sixty-nine separate Blue Shield plans. Dr. F. J. L. Blasingame, executive vice-president of the AMA, urged local Blue
Shield plans and state medical societies to cooperate in getting
the program underway, but it aroused little enthusiasm among
these groups. The plan would have provided full medical and
surgical payments for those whose incomes were below $2500
annually ($4000 for a couple). Participating physicians treat-
ing persons earning more than these amounts would receive the
same payments under the plan, but could then charge the patient whatever they wished in addition.

As in the past, the association emphasized its opposition to
governmental involvement, monetarily or otherwise, and the
insurance program was specifically identified as the AMA "answer" to proposals to "socialize" medicine. Moreover, the AMA
refused to endorse the earlier proposal advanced by the Blue

Cross Association to cover hospital fees. Their objection was to the use of government funds to pay the premiums for the needy. A spokesman for the hospital association charged that the AMA had even sought to prevent discussion of the proposal at the joint BCA-AHA meeting.[12]

Secretary of Health, Education, and Welfare, Abraham Ribicoff attacked the AMA plan on January 21, 1962 as completely inadequate, pointing out that it would do nothing to assist in the payment of costly hospital bills. He said, however, that it indicated that the AMA recognized that there was a problem, and called upon organized medicine to support the Administration program (which did not contemplate payment for physicians' bills) as a complement to its proposal. The AMA did not respond; apparently no response seemed necessary, since the defeat of the Javits amendment in July had settled the issue for that year. However, an angry President Kennedy appeared before television cameras on July 18, one hour after the crucial vote, to vow renewed efforts to pass a similar program in 1963.

On February 7, 1963, the President resubmitted his health proposals to the Congress and urged their speedy passage. On the same day, the AMA suggested that the problems could be solved by increased aid to the needy under the existing Kerr-Mills program. Both the Kennedy Administration and a group of Republican liberals introduced bills that would have provided for governmental health insurance; yet Congress took no action that year, despite the Administration's pressure. By 1964, however, the situation had changed considerably; not only was it a presidential election year, but there was a different occupant, Lyndon B. Johnson, in the White House. Supporters wondered whether these factors could produce action in the Congress, but they had little optimism.

Again, there were rival bills introduced by Administration supporters and by others. The health insurance industry was working feverishly to increase benefits and to extend coverage in an effort to demonstrate that there was no need for a governmental program. Health insurance executives conceded privately that, contrary to popular opinion, there has been considerable profit in providing insurance to the aged population.[13] The concerted effort was well underway in 1963 when many companies eliminated medical questions from their applications and engaged in intensive enrollment drives directed at those who were 65 and over. In their effort to avert a federal program, the industry then began providing opportunities for older persons to obtain insurance regardless of their age or physical condition, when shortly before there was no possibility whatever for many to procure it at a reasonable price.

The insurance companies made major gains. The Health Insurance Institute, an industry organization, estimated that at the end of 1963 there were 145 million Americans with hospitalization coverage, 3.6 million more than at the end of 1962, and more than triple the 42 million at the end of 1946. The institute estimated that of the 145 million, 135 million had some surgical protection, and 101 million some medical coverage. These figures exceed the estimates for the end of 1962 by 3.8 million for surgical coverage, and by 2.8 million for medical. The fastest growing form of coverage appeared to be major medical insurance.[14] However impressive these figures are, a Senate subcommittee charged that they were deliberate distortions. The Senate Subcommittee on the Health of the Elderly, under the chairmanship of Senator Pat McNamara (D-Mich.) issued a report on July 20 that maintained that three-fourths of the elderly lacked adequate hospital protection as defined by the American Hospital Association, that is, insurance providing for payment of 75 per cent of hospital costs. The report said that the better private health plans were prohibitively expensive. At a time when average charges for room and board in hospitals exceeded twenty dollars per day, the majority of policies provided for payment of ten dollars a day or less. The eight Democrats on the subcommittee endorsed the report; the four Republicans all rejected it, and the general manager of the Health Insurance Association of America took umbrage at its "unbalanced view."

President Johnson's "state-of-the-union Message" of January 8, 1964, called for governmental health insurance for older citizens to be financed through the social security system. On January 15, he spoke to a group of leaders from organizations supporting the health care effort, and asserted that he had "just begun to fight." Notwithstanding the pessimism of many key political leaders regarding the bill's chances for passage in 1964, the president placed it in a position of importance on his agenda of vital legislation, indicating that he considered it essential to victory in his "war on poverty." The AMA on January 9 immediately charged the President with "errors of fact," suggesting that his advisers had been supplying him with misinformation regarding the nature and cost of his own proposals and the need for any increase in governmental activity. Rather than being an "insurance" program, charged the AMA, it would be a "tax" program. The AMA spokesmen indicated that they had always favored helping those in need, but that such help already was available under the 1960 Kerr-Mills law. Administration officials had consistently criticized this law as inadequate because it is not in effect in every state, it requires the recipient of aid to have exhausted many of his financial resources before seeking assistance, and it requires the applicant to undergo a means test that many consider "degrading."

As had been the case for several years, the Administration-supported measure had been introduced in the House by Representative Cecil King (D-Calif.), and in the Senate by Senator Clinton P. Anderson (D-N.M.). On June 24, the slim hopes for passage of a health program were further reduced by the House Ways and Means Committee, when it set aside the King bill, and reported out a substitute bill that provided a raise in payments to social security beneficiaries but ignored the whole question of health care. Secretary of Health, Education, and Welfare Anthony Celebrezze expressed the fear that using a tax increase to finance an increase in benefit payments would put the prospects of a health program in great peril, since there seemed to be little room for further tax increases in the social security mechanism.

The Administration supporters in the Senate sought to effect a compromise. Senators Mike Mansfield (D-Mont.), Hubert Humphrey (D-Minn.), and Anderson sponsored a substitute measure—prepared by the former Secretary of Health, Education, and Welfare, under President Kennedy, Senator Abraham Ribicoff (D-Conn.) —that would offer social security beneficiaries the choice of a seven-dollar monthly benefit increase or a two-dollar increase plus health-care benefits. The health benefits would have provided ninety days of hospitalization with the patient paying for the first two and one-half days, or an option of forty-five days of hospitalization with no deductibles. Each option included coverage for a number of home health visits provided by certain agencies. The tax rate was to rise gradually from the current 3.625 per cent on the first $4800 dollars of wages paid by each the employee and the employer, to 5 per cent in 1971, to be paid on the first $5400. The bill provided for administration of the program by an agency that was not identified, but which was anticipated to be the Blue Cross Association. The Senate Finance Committee, however, dealt a blow to the Administration on August 17 by reporting out the social security measure without approval of any health care amendments.

In one last effort, the Senate supporters of health care attempted to attach provisions similar to the Ribicoff amendment to the social security bill during the floor debate. The crucial vote was set for September 2. Senator Barry Goldwater took time out from a busy campaign to fly back to Washington from Phoenix to vote against the amendment (he supported a proposal that would have raised benefits without adding health care). On a roll call of 49 to 44 the Senate adopted the amendment. Along with 44 Democrats, the measure received the votes of 5 liberal Republicans who, in return for their support, secured the adoption of an amendment allowing private insurance companies to pool their risks in order to offer relatively low-cost insurance as a supplement to the government plan, without fear of anti-trust action. The final vote on the bill, which came the next day, was 60 to 28 in favor.

For the first time in history, one house of Congress had acted favorably upon a bill calling for a general program of governmental health insurance. In the House-Senate Conference Committee, however, the House representatives refused to accept the health amendment, the Senate representatives refused to retreat from the Senate position, and the entire bill was killed. For the first time since 1952, there was an election year with no legislation improving or extending the social security system.

Supporters of the measure found one glimmer of hope in the results. Representative Wilbur Mills (D-Ark.) had long been the most powerful figure in the Congress in blocking any general health care plan; as chairaman of the House Ways and Means Committee he was in a position to forestall any favorable action. But on September 29, prior to the final rejection of the social security bill by the Conference Committee, Representative Mills announced: "I want to make it clear that I have always thought there was a great appeal in the argument that wage earners, during their working lifetime, should make payments into a fund to guard against the risk of financial disaster due to heavy medical costs." He hinted that he might support an alternative measure providing a Medicare fund separate from the social security trust fund. He hinted also that such a plan might be considered by his committee in 1965, and that it might provide for a system within the "private sector" of the economy, but this was not absolutely necessary.[15] In November, following President Johnson's landslide victory in the presidential election, Representative Mills said that he was ready to bring this bill before his committee if the President requested that he do so, but he reiterated his opposition to the plan as then formulated. But he was "acutely aware," as he had said publicly some time before, that there *was* a problem that had to be met.[16] An editorial in the *New York Times* charged that Mills had exercised a "one-man blockade" for four years against Medicare, and that he was largely responsible for the nation's having no program as of the end of 1964. It commented, however, that the magnitude of the President's victory apparently was having a "mellowing" effect.[17]

The new year 1965 began with a burst of health care activity. The thirteen-member Advisory Council on Social Security that Secretary Celebrezze had appointed in 1963 released its recommendations on January 2. The Council favored an extensive program of hospital care for the aged and the disabled, but one to be financed by a payroll tax separate from social security; there can be little doubt that this was done in order to win the approval of Wilbur Mills. The Council further recommended that the tax apply to the first $7200 of earnings, rather than the first $4800. A few days later, on January 6, a revised Anderson-King Bill was the first bill to be introduced into the Eighty-ninth Congress. In the Senate it carried the endorsement of forty-one co-sponsors, including three Republicans, Senators Kuchel (Calif.), Case (N.J.), and Javits (N.Y.). On January 7, the President sent a special message to Congress in which he proposed the creation of an extensive national health program that would include needy children as well as the aged. It gave first priority to Medicare, calling for a separate trust fund within the social security system. Representative Mills commented that the plan met his basic objections. All signs pointed toward overwhelming support for the measure.

The AMA leadership saw the need for a fresh approach if its efforts to defeat Medicare were again to be successful. Johnson's landslide victory in the presidential election and the strongly pro-Administration bent of the new Congress indicated that the association's earlier approach, so long successful, would no longer serve.

Accordingly, on January 9, organized medicine made a radical departure from tradition and proposed a health plan of its own that called for government subsidies to assist in providing health care to persons who were past the age of sixty-five, and who were in financial need. The AMA's president, Donovan Ward, said that the new proposal was merely a "redefinition" of policy which would be administered through the AMA-approved Kerr-Mills program and not through the social security system. The AMA called its plan "Eldercare." The proposal was announced to the "National Conference on Kerr-Mills," a gathering of representatives from state medical societies at the Sheraton-Chicago Hotel. It had been approved, not by the House of Delegates, the official policy-making body of the AMA, but by the board of trustees, the group that guides the activities of the organization between meetings of the House of Delegates.

Under the Eldercare plan, elderly persons would purchase private health insurance or nonprofit private prepayment coverage such as that provided by Blue Cross and Blue Shield plans, and would pay all or a part of the cost, depending upon their incomes. State governments, using their own funds plus federal grants, would pay part or all of the cost for those whose incomes were below certain limits. Dr. Ward said that the plan "would provide far more to our elderly citizens than is proposed in the Administration's medicare tax program. . . aid would consist of comprehensive health care benefits, rather than being limited to hospital and nursing home care representing only a fraction of the cost of sickness." Eldercare would also be superior to the Administration's plans according to the AMA spokesman, because it would operate within the established insurance system and be administered by private insurance companies and existing insurance and prepayment plans (such as Blue Cross); it would include drug, surgical, and medical costs not contemplated under the Medicare bill; and it would accomplish "far more" than Medicare "with none of the attendant evils of unpredictable expense, invasion of medical practice by the Federal bureaucracy, or disruption of the private health insurance industry by the Government."

Dr. Ward emphasized that in formulating its plan the AMA had consulted the American Hospital Association, the national Blue Cross and Blue Shield groups, the Health Insurance Association of America, and the American Dental Association—implying that Eldercare had the endorsement of those groups. However, spokesmen for the AHA and the Blue Cross Association made it known that the plan was solely that of the AMA and was not being co-sponsored by their groups. Further, the board of trustee's endorsement of Eldercare apparently came as a surprise to the leaders of local medical societies, many of whom, in a nation-wide poll, indicated that they were bewildered by the proposal and by AMA's seeming reversal of policy.[18]

On January 11, Senator Saltonstall (R-Mass.) and five other Republican senators introduced an alternative to the Administration plan that went beyond it in some respects, such as providing for some drugs and physicians' fees. On January 27, when the House Ways and Means Committee began its hearings on health care, Representative A. Sidney Herlong, Jr. (D-Fla.) introduced the Eldercare proposal in the House. He was joined in support of the bill by Representative Thomas B. Curtis (R-Mo.), the second-ranking Republican on the Ways and Means Committee, who had long been identified with AMA views. On the following day, the association officially endorsed the Herlong measure as the legislative embodiment of its Eldercare program.

The same day, prominent House Republicans introduced a health care plan of their own, supported by all the Republicans who were members of the Ways and Means Committee except Representatives Broyhill and Curtis (who, of course, exercised their influence in favor of the rival Herlong bill). The Republican plan introduced by Representative John W. Byrnes (R-Wisc.) was a voluntary program involving the pay-

ment of premiums by the beneficiary, the amount to depend
upon his ability to pay. Benefits were to be financed by the
premiums collected, supplemented by federal appropriations
as needed. All persons sixty-five and over would have been
eligible to participate, and would have received payment for
a maximum of forty thousand dollars of their lifetime health
expenses. The plan contemplated payment of the first one
thousand dollars of hospital and nursing home room and board
costs, and eighty percent of additional expenses.

By this time it was apparent that some kind of government
health plan was going to be enacted; both parties, in both
houses of Congress were strongly endorsing a variety of proposals—and even the AMA was sponsoring a plan that was
embodied in a bill that had been introduced. On March 10,
one of the last major impediments fell when Wilbur Mills issued an outright endorsement of the Administration's Medicare proposals. Less than two weeks later, on March 23, the
House Ways and Means Committee favorably reported the
Medicare bill, after having added liberalizing features that
even its sponsors would not have dared to suggest in previous
years, or even as late as the beginning of 1965. The measure
called for a 7 per cent increase in cash benefits to social security
beneficiaries, and included provisions for the payment of hospital and nursing home costs. Additionally there was a voluntary program calling for the payment of physicians' fees. This
aspect of the plan was based on the Byrnes proposal that had
received the support of leading House Republicans. The Committee had, for about three weeks, been considering ways in
which the features of the Administration bill and the Byrnes
plan could be combined. Immediately after the Committee reported the bill, President Johnson hailed the action and praised
the committee chairman, Representative Mills, for having re-
solved the difficulties. The vote in the committee was on a
straight party basis, seventeen Democrats in favor, and eight
Republicans opposed. The Committee did not vote on the
Herlong "Eldercare" bill, but it did vote on a plan for an en-

tirely voluntary program that was advanced by Representative Byrnes; the tally was two Democrats and eight Republicans in favor, fifteen Democrats opposed.[19]

Representative Byrnes testified at the hearings that it was unnecessary to consider the AMA-Herlong Eldercare Bill, since such a program could be placed into effect within the states under the provisions of either his bill or that of the Administration, since both bills would provide increased grants to states under the Kerr-Mills legislation. The Rules Committee cleared the bill for floor action on April 6 (nine Democrats and the California Republican H. Allen Smith in favor, four Republicans and the Mississippi Democrat William M. Colmer opposed). Amendments from the floor were prohibited.

On April 8, by vote of 313 to 115 the House approved the Administration's Medicare Bill after defeating the Byrnes substitute bill by a vote of 236 to 191; Representative Hale Boggs (D-La.), the majority whip, declared that it was the most important bill that had come before the Congress during his twenty-two years of service. For the first time, a House-approved health insurance program was on its way to the Senate Finance Committee for hearings. The hearings began on April 29, with Secretary Celebrezze as the first witness.

The secretary praised the measure, but criticized the House for having deleted coverage under the basic plan of the services of radiologists, pathologists, anesthesiologists, and specialists in physical medicine. He noted that such services are normally considered "hospital services" and billed as such. Thus his only criticism was a relatively minor one, considering the fact that the services mentioned would, in any event, be covered under the contemplated voluntary insurance plan that was to supplement the basic benefits.

Senator Russell Long (D-La.), the Senate Majority whip, the second ranking member of the Senate Finance Committee, and an opponent of Medicare in earlier sessions, reversed himself and on April 30 spoke in favor of governmental health insurance through social security. He criticized the bill, how-

ever, for not providing coverage for catastrophic illness, and
announced that he was drafting a substitute measure. Long's
bill, offered on May 18, proved to be a major obstacle to the
Administration's plan. Long wished to remove all limitations
on the amounts of hospitalization, nursing home, and home
health benefits provided, while making all benefits contingent
upon "ability to pay." Thus, there would be a sliding scale
of deductibles that the beneficiary would be required to pay
based upon his income. Senator Long's substitute would have
eliminated both the voluntary features of the supplement plan
and the requirement that participants in it pay a small monthly
premium. Under Long's plan, patients would pay ten per cent
of the costs of care above the deductible amount, but never an
amount in excess of fifty per cent of personal income. However,
the Senator announced that regardless of the fate of his amendment, he would support whatever program the Committee
might approve.

During its study the Committee adopted several minor
amendments, such as one providing coverage of certain spe-
cialized services received in a hospital that Secretary Celebrezze
had requested. On June 17, however, the Committee reversed
itself and adopted the Long amendment rather than the House-
approved program. This completely changed the emphasis of
the plan. Instead of providing general but limited benefits to
all, the plan favored by the Committee would have provided
unlimited benefits—but only to the needy. This setback to supporters of a general health plan was only temporary. On June
23, the Committee again reversed itself; it deleted the Long
amendment and restored the original program based upon the
Anderson-King approach. And on June 24, the Committee reported the bill favorably by a vote of 12 to 5. Ten Democrats
were joined by Republicans Everett Dirksen (Ill.) and Frank
Carlson (Kan.) in favor, and one Democrat (Harry Byrd of
Virginia) allied himself with the four Republicans in opposition.

The Medicare debate began on July 6, with Russell Long as

floor manager. Long said that the bill would be "the largest and most significant piece of social legislation ever to pass the Congress in the history of the country," and that he was unstinting in his praise for it. On July 7, by the narrow vote of 43 to 39, the senate defeated an amendment by Senator Ribicoff that would have removed the limitation on hospital care. After defeating all major amendments, the Senate finally approved the bill on July 9. The vote was an overwhelming sixty-eight in favor (fifty-five Democrats and thirteen Republicans) and twenty-one opposed (seven Democrats and fourteen Republicans).

The long journey was nearly complete. The Conference Committee cleared the bill on July 21, the House approved the Conference Committee report on July 27, and the Senate on July 28. The House vote was 307 to 116 (237 Democrats and 70 Republicans for, and 48 Democrats and 68 Republicans against), and the Senate vote was 70 to 24 (57 Democrats and 13 Republicans for and 7 Democrats and 17 Republicans against). All that remained was the signature of a President who had been strongly outspoken in support of the program, and on July 30, in the auditorium of the Truman Library in Independence, Missouri, and under the eye of the former President, Mr. Johnson provided that signature. In so doing he honored Harry S. Truman, the first American President to have sent the Congress a message devoted primarily to health care and requesting passage of appropriate laws—legislation that would have been considerably broader in scope than the Act finally passed twenty years later.

V

the rhetorical battle

Congress was largely silent on the health care question for some years following the election of Dwight D. Eisenhower to the presidency in 1952, but the issue again came into prominence with the introduction of the Forand Bill in 1957. It was debated even more heatedly after the election of John F. Kennedy in 1960. A major plank in Kennedy's platform was his firm support of such an amendment, and when the Medicare Bill was passed in 1965, the federal government was, in a sense, putting into effect a portion of the "Kennedy Program" that had remained as unfinished business in the years immediately following the assassination of the President; a portion that had, itself, been based on Forand's earlier efforts.

This chapter deals with the struggles by opponents and proponents of governmental health insurance to advance their points of view, beginning with the most intensive of all the campaigns, the one ending with the defeat of the Anderson-Javits amendment in 1962, and following to the present.

The battle over the Anderson-King bill was one in which each side took its case to the people by means of virtually every medium of mass communication—newspapers, magazines, radio, and television—and even sent prominent spokesmen into debate. The American Medical Association found its champion in the person of the chairman of its speakers bureau, Dr. Edward Annis. Almost singlehandedly Dr. Annis bore the burden of the association's speechmaking, giving voice to its message in all parts of the country, and often debating with proponents of the legislation such as Walter Reuther and Senator Hubert Humphrey. Annis also became "editor-at-large" of *Medical Economics,* a magazine devoted largely to the "business side" of medical practice and distributed by its publishers free of charge to physicians. A column bearing his by-line appeared in each bi-weekly issue, carrying accounts of how he managed to convince citizens who supported the bill (who spoke to him after having recognized him in a crowd, on an airliner, etc.) of the error of their ways.

Among Dr. Annis's many accomplishments was his election as president of the American Medical Association—the first president of the association in more than forty years who had not previously been a member of the House of Delegates, served on the Board of Trustees, or served on any of the councils and committees of the Association.[1]

Dr. Annis proved to be a clever spokesman, and under his leadership the American Medical Association continued to make effective use of the advice of public relations experts. On May 20, 1962, President Kennedy appeared as speaker at a televised rally in Madison Square Garden to call for support of the Anderson-King Bill. His Administration scheduled this as one of forty-two meetings accross the country to arouse favorable public reaction toward the program. The American Medical Association thereupon dispatched half of its "task force on the Anderson-King Bill," headed by Jim Reed, the association's director of communications, to New York to obtain paid radio-television time for a rebuttal and to handle relations with the press. The other half remained at the AMA's headquarters in Chicago to keep in touch with the association's executive director and its other key officials.[2] The very next night, Dr. Annis spoke from the same platform that had been used by President Kennedy. One hundred ninety television stations affiliated with the National Broadcasting Company carried his remarks to the public. The Garden, however, was empty—in striking contrast to the full and enthusiastic house welcoming Kennedy's address. Tom Hendricks, the assistant to the AMA's executive director, said that the Association could never have duplicated the appeal of the President of the United States in preparing for a meeting, so the public relations officials of the AMA deliberately decided upon a backdrop of empty seats for contrast.[3]

The National Broadcasting Company outlet in Boston refused to carry the American Medical Association rebuttal. The station's policy was to refuse to sell time to an organization to discuss controversial questions in which the organization was involved. The AMA charged that the station, which had carried Mr. Kennedy's telecast, was "blacking out" one side of a controversy in the President's home town. The allegation is similar to the frequent charge that the AMA carefully keeps from the pages of its publications any comments from physicians opposing its official views.

Mr. Hendricks listed several other measures planned in the AMA's campaign of opposition to the bill. In addition to more radio and television appearances by prominent physicians and others who favored the stand taken by the American Medical Association and the use of its "very strong" national speakers bureau ready to supply speakers to any group at any location, Mr. Hendricks included as a calculated part of the AMA's efforts a *Reader's Digest* article (June, 1962) by Representative Thomas B. Curtis (R-Mo.) a member of the House Ways and Means Committee. Hendricks also included a follow-up discussion with Curtis that was scheduled to appear on a television program sponsored by the *Digest*.[4]

Representative Curtis, one of the foremost opponents of health care under social security, maintained that he had studied the issue and reached his conclusions objectively and independently, animated by a desire to aid sound legislation, not to be a spokesman for any interest group. It is interesting, therefore, that the assistant to the American Medical Association's executive director knew in advance of Mr. Curtis' efforts, and considered them to be a part of the AMA's formal propaganda program.

The major efforts in support of the Anderson-King Bill were made by the Administration, the National Council of Senior Citizens for Health Care through Social Security (founded and directed by Aime Forand), the American Nurses Association, the National Association of Social Workers, the American Public Welfare Association, and a number of other social welfare and public health organizations.[5] The American Nurses Association reported considerable pressure from physicians to change its stand upon the measure, and charged that many nurses had been forced to resign from the association by their physician employers. The Association's Washington representative, Miss Julia Thompson, testified during the Ways and Means Committee's hearings on the bill that medical societies in no less than thirty-five states had sought to "pressure" nurses associations in those states to disavow the pro-King-Anderson stance of the national organization.[6]

Among the major organizations opposing the bill were the American Medical Association, almost all insurance companies (with the notable exception of Nationwide Insurance Company, which endorsed the bill strongly), the National Association of Manufacturers, the United States Chamber of Commerce, the National Association of Retail Druggists, and most other professional dental and medical organizations. Though officially opposing the bill, the Blue Cross Association and the American Hospital Association were more willing to compromise, and worked rather closely with the Administration in preliminary planning of the organization and administration of any program that might be adopted. Both organizations spent many hours in meetings with federal representatives who were also permitted to make numerous visits to hospitals and the administrative headquarters of several local Blue Cross plans.[7] In the 1961 Ways and Means Committee hearings, Blue

Cross and American Hospital Association opposition took the form first of urging that the bill not be passed until it became more evident that it was needed and, second, recommending changes that they believed would improve the bill if Congress should nevertheless insist upon passing it.

In general, both supporters and opponents based their arguments upon the same traditional concepts, symbols, and clichés. They talked endlessly of "compulsion," "socialism," "quality of care," the "health and financial condition" of the "senior citizens," the "fiscal nature" or "aspects" of the proposal, the program's "compatibility (or incompatibility) with American ideals" or with social security, the character of existing programs, the traditional organization of medical practice, and the alleged deficiencies of the British National Health Service.

Opponents of federally supported health care tend to regard "compulsion" in health and welfare matters as "un-American." They typically favor programs that are "voluntary" as more in keeping with the freedom and dignity of the individual. Most organizations opposing the Anderson-King Bill, and almost all its political opponents, professed their support of the social security system, yet the system obviously involves economic compulsion; most opponents supported the Kerr-Mills Medical Aid to the Aged program (many of them, of course, as a tactical maneuver aimed at preventing adoption of a broader plan). Opponents of Medicare tended to praise Kerr-Mills as "voluntary," but both programs involve support from funds acquired through compulsory taxation, and neither requires patients or suppliers of health services to seek service or to render it.

Other factors were involved in the debate over the relative merits of the Anderson-King versus the Kerr-Mills plans (for example, the "state rights" issue and the whole question of "means tests"). The mere existence of compulsion seems to offer little explanation for most of the opposition; it appears to be hardly more than one of the many rhetorical devices employed by the disputants to bolster their own stands.

Proponents of the idea of health care through social security spoke of "compulsion" as a "necessary evil." But actually, they pointed out, only the tax was compulsory. This being so, was it not inconsistent to oppose Anderson-King because it involved "compulsion" while at the same time supporting the Medical Aid to the Aged program (Kerr-Mills), which was not only no less "compulsory" in regard to taxation but also allowed the several states to put severe restrictions on the sources from which patients under the program might receive their health services? In admitting that the Anderson-King program would involve compulsion, its partisans averred that *all* programs supported by taxation are compulsory. Further, what would be compelled by Anderson-King would be compulsory "insurance" analogous to the compulsory insurance required of most people by the 1935 Social Security Act. And insurance, whereby individuals provide for their own future, is truly "American"— as everyone knows.

The term "socialism" is sufficiently imprecise to be almost meaningless even when those using it wish to discuss matters rationally. As used in the course of the health care controversy, the word lost whatever meaning it had possessed before. It was often used but seldom defined, and such definitions as were attempted were not calculated to lend clarity to the discussions. "Social welfare services," "compulsory health insurance," "government ownership of health facilities with physicians on the government payroll," "a regimental system of state health care precluding all professional freedom for practitioners and all freedom of choice for patients"—such were a few of the many and disparate explanations of "socialism" that were commended to the attention of the American public.

Though there were hardly two persons who could agree on what it was, virtually everyone who talked or wrote favorably or unfavorably about Medicare expressed unwavering hostility to "socialism." Opponents sought to show that the program provided for by the Anderson-King bill was in itself socialistic or was, at the very least, the "entering wedge" or the "foot-in-the-door," and would inevitably become socialism. Those favorable to the bill seemed equally intent on proving that the program was not socialistic and would not lead to socialized medicine. All parties to the Anderson-King debate agreed tacitly to reject any program that they could agree was "socialistic."

The agreement to reject "socialism" had no significant effect on events, however, since any program would be, and often was, called socialistic by opponents or defended as non-socialistic by its supporters, with all concerned citing the same facts and using the same "logical" processes. Thus, adherents of contradictory positions tended to accept the same basic values and presuppositions and went on to define their positions accordingly; that is, they accepted the relevance of the same symbols, with the result that their ideological orientations, if not identical, were, at least on the surface, strikingly similar.

It is possible that the antagonists recognized the nonsense inherent in the hysterical debate over "socialism" and cynically used the term to influence public opinion on the emotional level. But it is surely neither profitable nor necessary to question motives in this instance; the question of intent is immaterial. Whether we grant the sincerity of those arguing the question of socialism, or charge that they all attempted to arouse favorable responses while deliberately concealing the fundamental elements of the issue, the fact remains that both parties to the controversy tended to accept certain symbols as relevant, and both parties used them to support positons that were flatly contradictory. Though there was probably some hypocrisy involved, many on both sides seem to have believed with complete sincerity in the relevancy of their views on socialism to the Medicare debate.

The opponents of the Kennedy Administration's health care proposals employed tactics essentially identical to those that had been used in the Whitaker and Baxter campaign during President Truman's administration. Physicians resumed the distribution of leaflets and reprints of magazine articles to their patients and others. Doctors' offices were decorated with large

posters headed "Socialized Medicine and You" with a text similar to that of the leaflets.

A typical example entitled "An Important Message from Your
Doctor," stresses compulsion and governmental control and
charges that the program would "place a third party—Washington bureaucrats—between the patient and the physician. It
would place politics at the bedside of the ill." Not only would
the patient's "free choice of hospital and physician" be limited,
but the bill "would eliminate the privacy of the patient-physi-
cian relationship . . . making it possible for government clerks
to examine the most intimate personal health records—records
that are now a private matter between patient and physician."
Or, it may be observed, between patient, physician, insurance-
company clerks, physicians' aides, hospital workers, etc. This
leaflet varies the socialism charge, saying merely that the program would be the "first step toward socialized medicine in this
country . . . a system that has resulted in the deterioration of
medical care wherever it has been tried." It ends by expressing
the hope that those who agree will convey their thoughts to
their Congressmen. "Working together, we can preserve the
high quality of medical care now available in this country. Let's
keep politics out of medicine."

A leaflet entitled "It's *Your* Decision" assures readers that
organized medicine does favor " . . . a *voluntary* program . . . .
voluntary health insurance for those able to purchase it and
the Kerr-Mills Law for helping those who need help in paying
for medical care." However, lest the patient imagine that "socialized medicine" is not at issue, it declares: "And we are not
crying 'wolf' when we apply that term to the Anderson-King
Bill now before Congress." The bill, with its limited services,
its compulsion, its deleterious effect on the quality of care, its
expense, its inequity—the Anderson-King Bill "would mean
socialized health care . . . immediately for all those over 65 eligible for Social Security and eventually for every man, woman,
and child in America." Again, patients who agreed with their

doctor that a "Federal Government-controlled health care scheme for any segment of our population would be bad for the nation" were urged to write to their representatives in Congress.

These arguments were disseminated not only in leaflets and posters but also in the mass communication media. In concert with local medical societies and other sympathetic organizations, the American Medical Association throughout the country flooded the newspapers with advertisements similar to the leaflets.

In New Mexico, for example, the Chaves County Medical Society placed an advertisement in the *Roswell Daily Record* (May 27, 1962). This advertisement, which was endorsed by the District No. 5 Association of Registered Nurses, the Chaves County Pharmaceutical Association, and the Roswell Dental Society, asked—and purportedly answered—the question: "Can governments doctor? President Kennedy and his associates say YES. We, your physicians, say NO. BUT, this is more than a medical issue. It is an issue affecting not only the health of our people, but the economic and political freedom of our country." It called the plan obviously inadequate and charged that its proponents had "relied upon showmanship, emotionalism, invective, and innuendo," to sell this plan to the American people. "We believe their real reasons for wanting this legislation so badly have never been stated honestly and openly," it continues, illustrating what Richard Hofstadter has termed the "paranoid style" in American politics.[8] Morever, "any legislation, which through its immediate, or its potential effect, further reduces man to the nameless subservience of the welfare state, is a disavowal of the very concepts upon which this nation was founded. This is such a plan."

The advertisement cites the Declaration of Independence to the effect that it is the right and the duty of men to throw off a government when the government "evinces a design to reduce them under absolute despotism"; the apparent implication being that, if the Anderson-King Bill were passed, the "people"

should "throw off" the federal government.[9] The advertisement goes on to list a number of reasons for the society's opposition to the bill, and declares that the society has unanimously
endorsed resolutions condemning the program passed by the
AMA's House of Delegates.

In New York state, the Medical Society of the county of
Monroe placed a similar advertisement in the *Rochester Democrat* (April 25, 1962). It included the arguments against compulsion, against cost, and against permitting hospital, nursing
home, and physicians' services to be "brought under control of
a federal bureaucrat in Washington" where political decisions
would "determine the operations of our outstanding Rochester
hospitals!" It then listed the limitations of the proposal's coverage and benefits, and saved as its final argument: "It is *not*
prepayment and it is not insurance and the people who receive
the service will not have paid for it!"

A similar advertisement in a Pennsylvania paper, the *Harrisburg Patriot* (May 18, 1962), sponsored by the Dauphin County Medical Society, prompted editorial comment on the "Doctors' Scare Campaign." According to the *Patriot* editorial, the
American Medical Association "has gone far beyond noise and
occasional exaggeration. The very heart of what it is saying to
the public is a calculated attempt to distort the meaning of
the bill and to play on fears. For this reason it is sad to see the
Dauphin County Medical Society, in a message signed, 'Your
Doctor,' echoing this line to residents of the Harrisburg area."

These and other advertisements were not merely consistent
with the American Medical Association propaganda effort, but
were apparently based largely, if not entirely, upon material
supplied directly by the association. In New Mexico, in New
York, in Pennsylvania, in virtually every state, local and regional organizations expressed the same thoughts and used the
same propaganda techniques—often the same language—as the
national organization.

The American Medical Association's own advertisement appeared in newspapers throughout the country. Typical was the

one that appeared in the *New York Times* (April 19, 1962),
and in some thirty-five other widely dispersed metropoli-
tan newspapers. It began: "Speaking for 180,000 physician-
members . . . the American Medical Association believes you
deserve to know exactly where we doctors stand on the question of MEDICAL AID for the AGED." Though this advertisement went into more detail than most locally sponsored ones,
the format ("here's what we favor—here's what we reject") was
essentially the same.

Coupled with the American Medical Association's newspaper
campaign was a concurrent one on radio. In order to reach
the "opinion leaders" of the nation, the Association placed
many announcements on FM radio also, since FM program-
ming often is directed to a "select" radio audience.

When Medicare's opponents mentioned the related issues of
"socialism" and compulsion, they usually charged that the bill,
in spite of the section prohibiting federal interference with
hospitals or with the practice of medicine, would severely restrict the free choice by the patient of physician and hospital.
The basis for this was that the program would pay for services
rendered only in institutions having agreements with the federal
government; if the patient's physician happened not to have
staff privileges at such a hospital, the patient would have to
seek services of another physician who would be able to admit
him. The same restriction on freedom of choice obtains without
a program of federal health benefits. If a patient desires admission to a certain hospital, he is limited in his choice of physician to one permitted to practice in that hospital; conversely,
if the patient wishes to receive care from the physician of his
choice, he is limited to the hospital selected by that physician,
and the physician is limited in his selection to the few hospitals
in which he may practice. This system, by which hospitals select those physicians who are permitted to use their facilities, is
justified by the need to maintain the quality of medical practice
within the hospital; but, at the same time, it enables physicians
to restrict the professional activities of other physicians on

grounds having nothing to do with professional competence. Thus, if a local medical society succeeds in persuading hospitals in the vicinity to deny staff privileges to a certain physician it becomes extremely difficult for him, without access to a hospital, to continue to practice medicine. The drafters of the bill, in addition (deliberately avoiding the term "standards" as political anathema implying coercion), drew the "conditions of participation" for hospitals so that all but those that were markedly substandard could qualify. Those accredited by the Joint Commission on Accreditation of Hospitals, a substantial number, could qualify virtually automatically.

Other factors, such as the ability of the patient to pay and his geographic location, also influence the present range of freedom of choice. Wayne Menke, a careful student of the cultural implications of American medical practice, observes that "one of the standard arguments against compulsory insurance is that it would restrict the patient's free choice of physician. But how this choice would be restricted under compulsory insurance to a greater degree than it is now restricted by other factors is not entirely clear. So obvious are the factors of distribution and economics under the present system that some have argued that there might actually be more freedom of choice under compulsory insurance." [10] In any event, the allegation that the program would restrict the patient's freedom of choice seems, at best, to be ill-founded.

Closely associated with the "freedom of choice" issue, by both supporters and opponents of the Anderson-King Bill, was the question of its effect on the quality of health care. Opponents often argued that governmental payment for health services would result in "assembly-line" or "G. I." medicine, and that the public would abuse the system, seeking hospital care when not really necessary simply because it would be "free." The Anderson-King Bill sought to discourage overutilization of hospital services, indicating agreement in principle that there was danger of abuse. It specified that participating hospitals were to have utilization committees to ascertain whether facilities were used wisely and economically, and it provided for deductibles (the payment by the patient of ten dollars for the first nine days in a hospital during a "benefit period," with a minimum of twenty dollars for each period) to discourage unnecessary admissions or unnecessarily extended stays.

The major purpose of the deductible provision was to reduce costs to the government, but many supporters in Congress hailed the deductibles as safeguards against malingerers. Whether justified or not, both supporters and opponents tended to agree that recipients of services generally should not obtain them without some payment. This implies a suspicion that the public needs supervision to prevent it from hoarding any service or commodity provided on the basis of "something for nothing." This is not to pass judgment on that viewpoint, but merely to point out that many supporters shared it with opponents; the difference tended to be one of degree, not kind. The congressional supporters who accepted the proposition thought that the bill's restrictions controlled it adequately; the opponents denied it. Some of the bill's supporters opposed the deductibles, but were unable to have that provision removed. Opponents, on the alert for arguments favorable to their position, sometimes charged the majority of the supporters with inconsistency because of their support for deductibles. The American Hospital Association, officially an opponent of the program, recommended that if it were adopted it should be without deductibles. This was not purely the result of altruism, since the association recognized that without deductibles, hospitals would be assured of receiving the full amount owed them by the government, but must expect a certain loss on sums owed by private patients.

With extremely rare exceptions, all participants in the health-care controversy accepted the American Medical Association's estimate of the health service its members and other American physicians supply as being of the highest quality in the world. Arguing from this premise, opponents of the Anderson-King Bill charged that "socialism" in other countries is responsible for the poor quality of health care there as compared with that in the United States. The only data used to any extent to bolster the boastful estimate of the quality of American health care were the numbers of foreign physicians who seek training in the United States and the relatively large ratio of physicians in the United States to the general population.

Many experts have raised serious questions regarding several aspects of American health care. Herbert Ratner, M. D., director of public health for Oak Park, Illinois, and associate clinical professor of preventive medicine and public health at the Stritch School of Medicine of Chicago's Loyola University, has remarked that "there are a number of striking paradoxes that characterize American medicine, and they can be attributed to our failure to develop and maintain a sound, dynamic philosophy of medicine, and to teach and to practice medicine in the light of it. . . . One is that though the United States is the best place in the world in which to have a serious illness (because with our technical talents we have developed a high level of competency in handling complicated, serious illnesses), it is one of the worst countries in the world in which to have a nonserious illness." Asked why this is so, he said that "as actionists, who feel more comfortable doing something and having something done to us, we impose our life-saving drugs and techniques, intended for serious ailments, on minor, even trivial, illnesses—illnesses that are self-limited and that, except for occasional symptomatic relief, do better without interference from the physician. It is generally recognized that America is the most over-medicated, most over-operated, and most anxiety-ridden country with regard to health." [11]

Consumer Reports, in an article titled "Does the U. S. Really Have the World's Finest Medical Care?" quotes another medical educator as saying that though Americans have some of the best medical care in the world, we have also some of the worst. He asserts that we talk more about quality of care than do the Europeans, but that we do less about it.[12] The article presents several statistics that are unfavorable to American medicine:

England has lower death rates at every age up to sixty-five, half of the American draft rejectees have failed the physical tests, and the United States is a poor eleventh among nations with regard to the rate of infant mortality. It discusses a research project at the University of North Carolina that involved a close study of the practices and techniques of a sample of North Carolina physicians in which it was found that nearly half of them—judged by minimum and not unreasonably high standards—were substandard in at least one aspect of their performance. The article notes that "it has been clear for many years that there are serious quality problems in surgery."

Certainly the quality of American medical care as a whole is high. Reports such as those cited concentrate upon weaknesses and ignore strengths, and there are obvious problems concerning the use of comparative statistics. It is apparent, however, that neither the opponents of governmental health insurance nor its supporters have justified their sanguine attitude with regard to the American health care situation.

Even if it were possible to assess with any degree of precision the relative quality of health care in various nations, the issue is obviously irrelevant. The contention by Medicare's opponents that the United States, with its vast material resources, has a high quality of health care simply because of its organization of medical practice and its manner of paying physicians can hardly be taken seriously if examined objectively. Yet both opponents and proponents, the one explicitly and the other implicitly, spoke as though any change in medical practice would lower the quality of care. The arguments, therefore, centered not upon the desirability of the present system but upon whether the proposal would change it. Supporters stressed their view that the only change would be in the source of funds paying the bill. This implies either an acceptance of the dogma that any revision of the laissez faire fee-for-service medical system would be deleterious to the quality of care, or a belief that no program changing the system would be accepted. In either case the result is the same: arguments on both sides of the controversy were illustrated by similar concepts and symbols.

So much has been written regarding the health and financial condition of the aged and the fiscal soundness of the health-care program, that there is no need to discuss these issues in detail here. There is a proliferation of articles on these subjects, and the most convenient source for an overview of the pertinent issues is the four-volume report of the 1961 hearings before the Ways and Means Committee, *Health Services for the Aged Under the Social Security Insurance System.*

Opponents of the bill tended to minimize the economic difficulties of the aged, saying that those over sixty-five "in many respects . . . are better off than any other age group," as the American Medical Association asserted in its leaflet "25 Vital Questions and 25 Factual Answers on Health Care for the Aged." Supporters of governmental action pointed to the low income of the aged and the impossibility of their recovering financially following a severe drain on their economic resources. They called attention to the more frequent hospital admissions and the longer stays of the elderly. Some opponents responded by saying that as a rule the health picture of the aged is good, and there are no specific diseases of the aged; there are simply diseases among the aged. Supporters maintained that the bill would establish a fiscally sound program based on the "tried and true" principles of social security, but opponents believed that it would be too expensive, would not provide an adequate financial base, and would thereby endanger the soundness of the social security system itself.

Many opponents objected to the departure from the "tried and true" social security principle of cash benefits instead of services. Some of the more vociferous critics in Congress, the AMA, and the insurance industry used their opposition to health benefits to launch an attack upon the whole of the social security system, saying that it is itself fiscally unsound, and that its principles are not "tried and true" since the system has been in existence less than thirty years and has not yet matured. They continued to charge, moreover, that social security is not "really insurance," as though this were a crowning argument.

To some extent this is the heart of the issue. The antagonists expended great amounts of energy debating whether social security is actually insurance or not, the implication of both sides being that the value of the system depends to some degree on its meeting the definition of insurance. Supporters admitted that it is different from private insurance, but said that it may accurately be described as "social insurance." Both antagonists again displayed an acceptance of the same basic orientation while adopting contradictory positions. They reconciled the positions they adopted largely by rhetoric.

One other source of dispute was the adequacy of existing measures for assisting the aged to meet their health needs. The opponents of federal action usually said that the rapidly expanding health insurance industry, combined with the Kerr-Mills provisions and other programs, could meet the needs of the aged satisfactorily if only given a chance to do so. They pointed out that although the Kerr-Mills plan involves federal financing, it involves governmental administration more at state or local levels than from Washington. They inferred from this that the program could provide more adequately for varying conditions from one location to the next than could a federally-administered plan.

Supporters and opponents agreed on the basic statistics concerning health insurance coverage, but they disagreed on such fundamental issues as the adequacy of the coverage. Also, supporters replied to the allegation that the Kerr-Mills program was adequate by saying that many states had not adopted it, and, of those that had, many had placed such restrictions upon benefits that they were virtually worthless. The Kentucky version, for instance, provided hospitalization only for "acute, emergency, and life-endangering illness," and limited the period for which hospital benefits were provided to six days.[13]

The opponents responded that the Kerr-Mills Act permitted unlimited benefits and that it was up to the states to implement it. They charged that the Department of Health, Education, and Welfare discouraged states from accepting the provisions of the Act by using devious methods in order to strengthen the case for Medicare. The Department, of course, strenuously denied this.

Another basic divisive issue between supporters and opponents of the Anderson-King approach was the desirability of some test of the financial means of those seeking benefiits. Supporters argued that the means test is an affront to human dignity; opponents defended it as closely akin to a commercial credit check.

Both the Republican and Democratic parties tended to accept the principles of private medical practice combined with governmental action to aid a specific group, such as the aged or the needy aged. With the change from the Anderson-King Bill to the Anderson-Javits Amendment, the supporters even made concessions to non-federal administration and to the greatest possible use of private insurance companies—thereby incorporating more of the symbols of private enterprise into the proposed federal program. This proposed Anderson-Javits Amendment to H. R. 10606, the Public Welfare Amendments of 1962, included language ostensibly allowing Blue Cross administration and a private insurance option, both with little substance. The program as finally passed in 1965 retains a similar provision for private administration; that is, private organizations may serve as the channels through which payments are provided to institutions supplying health care.

Both political parties also tended to accept limitations upon the benefits to be provided. Opponents generally argued that the services contemplated were too costly to materialize and that even so they would be too limited to be of great value. They therefore advocated limitation of the population covered rather than limitations of services; thus, they would have lim-

ited the benefits of such a program to the needy aged. Supporters, on the other hand, usually seemed to accept limitations
upon the benefits as a positive good, evidently believing that
certain exclusions such as physicians' fees somehow prevented
the program from being "socialized medicine." The supporters
withdrew from this position to a degree, but not entirely, when
they were strong enough to enact the Medicare bill. Then they
supported payment for physicians' fees, but only on an optional
basis, and only with monthly "premiums" from the beneficiary.

Here again the antagonists expended considerable energy
upon essentially minor issues. When supporters pointed with
pride to the exclusion of physicians' services, the opponents
tended to say "Not so," referring to the coverage of the services
of interns and residents in training in hospitals, and to the
services of radiologists, anesthesiologists, physiatrists (specialists in physical medicine), and pathologists when rendered as
hospital services. The drafters of the bill simply followed accepted procedure in providing for the payment of the hospital
bill, but not the medical bill. This is the Blue Cross arrangement, which excludes the services of physicians, except when
their services are those traditionally offered as hospital services,
and leaves the medical bills to Blue Shield. Many specialty
groups have protested having their services covered under Blue
Cross rather than Blue Shield in an effort to emphasize their
professional autonomy and to secure the generally higher fees
that result from private billing as opposed to hospital payment.
Though they have sometimes succeeded in obtaining Blue
Shield, rather than Blue Cross, coverage for their services, there
is ample precedent for including them in the hospital bill. It
is interesting to note, just prior to the passage of Medicare,
Ways and Means Committee Chairman Wilbur Mills (D-Ark.),
a long time foe and belated supporter of the program, successfully fought to eliminate coverage for specialists' services under the basic hospitalization plan because of fears that it would
in some way encourage "socialized medicine."

The Keystone to the Arch

A major portion of the opponents' campaign against the Anderson-King Bill was, oddly enough, devoted to criticism of Great Britain's National Health Service. Generally speaking, the Administration's supporters did not respond to the allegations that the British system is a failure. The dissension lay mainly in the resemblance of the proposed program to that in Great Britain, with supporters saying that the systems had no similarity and opponents charging that the Administration's bill either would establish such a system here or would lead to its establishment. Though very few attempted to define "socialism," most agreed that the term applied to the National Health Service. This meant, therefore, that the value of the President's program depended somewhat upon its resemblance to the system in Great Britain—if at all similar, it would be "socialism" and bad. Only if it were determined to be clearly different in character from the British system could it be examined solely on its merits.

The discussion of the British National Health Service was an obvious attempt to add some substance to the term "socialism" and to increase its emotional connotations by supplying specific examples of the allegedly deleterious effects of "governmental medicine." Seldom did anyone undertake to examine the British system, since the tendency was to consider it merely "socialism," thereby classifying it as undesirable by definition. But the opponents used extreme arguments to associate the allegedly disastrous National Health Service with the proposal to add health benefits for the aged to the American social security system.

Other conservative organizations such as the Young Americans for Freedom added their efforts to those of the American Medical Association, the U. S. Chamber of Commerce, and the National Association of Manufacturers in opposing Medicare.[14] They frequently condemned the organization of health care in other countries, and built a campaign of opposition relying heavily upon the notion of an internal conspiracy. An example of opinion from the far right is the pamphlet "Tax Fax No. 35," published by the *Independent American,* describing itself as a national newspaper for conservatives dedicated to "restoring" constitutional government.[15] The pamphlet is entitled "Medicare, a Socialist Fraud" and subtitled "Importing England's Failure" and "Political Witch Doctors Plan Tax Increase to Finance Socialized Medicine." Under the heading "Socialist-Communist Backing" is the statement that it is no surprise that any proposal granting a role in medicine to the federal government receives support from socialists and communists. This "Socialist-Communist" label subsequently becomes "liberal-socialist," equating liberals not only with socialists but with communists as well.

Under the heading " 'Medicare' is Socialized Medicine" are references to denials from President Kennedy that the program would be socialistic and remarks that he considered a denial necessary because of his awareness that Americans believe "unvarnished socialism" to be distasteful. Representative Bruce Alger (R-Texas), an arch-conservative from Dallas (since defeated for re-election), is cited to refute Mr. Kennedy and to define the proposal as socialism. Government intrusion into personal lives is said to be the issue at stake.

The argument then turns to the limitations of the bill which are used as the basis for inferring a conspiracy. There allegedly are "devious stratagems" by which the "liberal-socialists" are able to "ram" legislation through Congress, and, the pamphlet asserts, it is clear that the drafters of the Anderson-King Bill deliberately included "so-called inequities" to restrict congressional debate to the provisions of the bill rather than its principles and those of socialized medicine. (Judging from the congressional debates, if such a conspiracy existed it was singularly unsuccessful.) The very principle of compromise is called a socialist tool. The federal grants that supplement state funds in Kerr-Mills programs, for example, come from appropriations to the Department of Health, Education, and Welfare. Thus, goes the reasoning, by their willingness to compromise, "so-called conservatives" in Congress enabled the federal government already to have a foot-in-the-door in the "field of federal interference" with medicine. Elsewhere, speaking of federal taxes, the leaflet by a strange twist says that such confiscation of the results of a man's labor must be called "National Socialism."

Under the headings "It Failed in England" and "No Freedom of Choice," the pamphlet devotes almost one-fourth of its space to an attack on the system in Great Britain. Its allegations are approximately the same as those by the business and professional organizations attacking the Anderson-King program.

Departing from the political fringes, it is interesting to note the character of the attack upon the British system by the American Medical Association and the National Association of Manufacturers. A leaflet dated November 1961, published by the NAM, and entitled "Medical Care Under Social Security" replies to the question, "Would the quality of medicine be enhanced by such a system?" by referring to health care in Britain as "bogged down in red tape and inefficiency." It quotes a former British physician who now resides in the United States and has traveled throughout the country speaking for the AMA as describing the "waste and regimentation of their system" and ends its answer by saying, "Our voluntary system of medical care is the best in the world—without government intrusion. Medicare for the aged under Social Security would be the first step along the road to a tragic duplication of Britain's mistake." The leaflet also makes the charge, repeated frequently by critics of the Administration's bill, that "there are *three* medical *clerks* for every *doctor*. On an equivalent basis here the U. S. government would have to hire nearly 2,000,000 more clerks!"

A pamphlet widely distributed by the AMA and individual physicians, "A Case Against Socialized Medicine," opens with the statement: "No one denies that Americans enjoy the best medical care in the world, but the quality of medical care physicians can offer their patients in the future depends upon the ultimate outcome of federal legislation now pending in Congress." It charges that the Anderson-King bill would mean socialized medicine for one part of the population and that eventually it would result in "socialized medicine for everyone." After saying that government medicine has been tried and found wanting, it points to Great Britain where costs were greater than anticipated, and calls hospital conditions there "deplorable." There follows a list of twenty-two brief quotations from British sources criticizing the National Health Service.

Another pamphlet, "Health Care U.S.A.," [16] carries on its cover a Norman Rockwell painting of a homely scene depicting an obviously robust little boy openly admiring the fatherly physician who has just taken a reading of his temperature. It discusses the painting in terms of the intangible bond between the American physician and his patient that cannot be communicated effectively by words, only by pictures. It notes that one of the nation's best-known artists has illustrated so well the warm relationship between a small boy and his family physician, and says that the same relationship exists between the American citizen and the other members of the "Healthcare, U.S.A. team," who, similar to the family physician, have devoted themselves to the relief of human misery. The pamphlet briefly mentions nursing homes, dental care, hospitals, health insurance including Blue Cross and Blue Shield, and the "captain" of the Healthcare, U.S.A. Team, the physician ("every team has to have a Captain"). It pays tribute to all members of the "team," and concludes that "Americans are world champions."

Rather than continuing this attitude of boastful exuberance, however, it modulates deftly into an attack upon other methods of organizing health care. In Soviet Russia, says a physician who spent two weeks there, the hospitals are far inferior to ours and we are three to four years ahead of the Russians in heart

surgery. Moreover, he says, there have been no great pharmaceutical research achievements in the USSR. In Manitoba, On-
tario and in New Zealand, costs are rising at alarming rates. In
Germany the availability of medical services without cost seems
to promote a demand for them. In France, though admittedly
the national health service has made hospital care generally
available, it has somehow prevented the development of good
hospital service! In Poland, religious organizations have developed health plans of their own and are drawing criticism from
the country's "organized atheists." The space devoted to Great
Britain's system is almost as great as that devoted to the others
combined, and the text duplicates the standard charges. Printed
across the bottom of the page is a quotation attributed to Lenin, "Compulsory Medicine is the keystone to the arch of Socialism." Incidentally, according to reference specialists in the
Library of Congress, this quotation cannot be found in any of
Lenin's writings.

Though the British National Health Service and its degree of
success or failure had no connection with the question of health
benefits through social security, the criticisms of the British
system that opponents used to attack the social security proposal became so extreme that the British Information Services, an
agency of the British Government, issued a rebuttal.[17] The
British explained that they were called upon to defend the
Health Service not to "sell" it to other countries, but "to correct misrepresentations deliberately put about." They said that
"falsehoods and half-truths about 'NHS' are sometimes spread
abroad by people who are campaigning against any governmental intervention in the medical and hospital services of
their own countries."

The release cites those most frequently heard criticisms
which it says are misrepresentations, and attempts to correct
them. It charges that the former British physician referred to
above, for example, supported his case "with statements that
are, to say the least, inaccurate." It says that his experience
under the Service was so limited that "his judgments on it

should be treated with caution. . . ." As to the allegation that
there are three clerks for each physician, it says that "this statement is utterly wrong and misleading" and that, of over 600,000
employees of the National Health Service, only about 4,000
are "administrative and clerical civil servants employed in the
Government Health Departments" plus some 40,000 in the hospital service or offices of local executive councils.

The reply from the British government was not the only
voice from Great Britain criticizing the statements of those opponents of social security health benefits who bolstered their
arguments by castigating the National Health Service. On September 15, 1961, Robert P. Varley, the rector of St. Peter's Epis-
copal Church in Salisbury, Maryland, presented "a highly emotional talk" to the semiannual meeting of the Medical and
Chirurgical Faculty of Maryland (the state medical society).[18]
He "called upon physicians to unite to resist socialistic influences in the United States, as represented by such men as 'the
Hoffas, the Reuthers and the Kennedys'." He charged that socialism in England has produced a climate in which it is no
longer an honor to be either a physician or a priest of the
Church of England. Mr. Varley, a member of the speakers bureau of the American Medical Association, was traveling in this
capacity to speak to medical societies in thirty-six states, and
testified similarly before the House Ways and Means Committee during the hearings on health benefits through social security. His testimony, again, was highly emotional and was punctu-
ated with charges of "socialism." When Representative King
questioned him in this regard, he hedged by saying that he
could not document his charges without undertaking the difficult task of defining "socialism"!

An editorial in the Baltimore *Sun* took his statements calmly,
mentioning that Mr. Varley was no physician but was a member
of the American Medical Association's speakers bureau who
called upon physicians in "emotional and politically rather
partisan terms" to fight "collectivism," and who seemed to
equate "governmental incursions into medical care with god-

lessness. Look, he said, at England." Less calm was the reaction from Great Britain. Mr. Varley was quickly and "strongly denounced by authoritative members of both callings in London." [19]

Subsequently, in an editorial entitled "AMA Versus NHS," the *British Medical Journal,* the journal of the British Medical Association, said that it was confident that many physicians in the United States "deplore, as we do, the vulgarity and cheapness of the AMA's past and present attacks upon the National Health Service." [20] It said that attempts to depict the British system as "socialized medicine" were a cover "to distract attention from the weaknesses of American medicine" and pointed out that "socialized medicine" is a term "whose exact meaning no one has yet defined." The *Journal* recalled that "three years ago, when *AMA News* published some nonsense about the NHS," it had suggested that the AMA should "find out how far American medicine falls behind in its service to the great American public" but that the "AMA still prefers to distract attention from the weaknesses of American medicine by hammering away at Britain's NHS."

The *Journal* cites the AMA leaflet, "A Case Against Socialized Medicine," and its three cartoons denouncing the British system, as being efforts of which it hopes "the AMA is heartily ashamed." "We do not recall," it says, "that those who favoured the introduction of the NHS buttressed their case by distorted propaganda against such abuses as American doctors themselves have admitted—fee-splitting, over-charging, unnecessary operations, sending patients to 'physician-owned drug stores', and so forth."

The emotionalism surrounding the health-care issue became so extreme as to cause markedly unfavorable public reaction and, in at least one case, an equally emotional response. In Point Pleasant, New Jersey, a group of physicians on the staff of the Point Pleasant Hospital signed a statement prepared by Dr. Bruce Henriksen beginning, "We, the undersigned . . . do refuse to participate in the care of patients under the provisions of the King-Anderson bill or similar legislation." New Jersey's Governor Hughes denounced the statement as a "political device"; and Secretary of Health, Education, and Welfare Ribicoff said that it was a "shocking" attempt to "blackmail the Congress and the American people." [21] An editorial in the Trenton *Evening Times* called it a "strange statement" and said that it "introduces a threat by a group of New Jersey physicians to ignore sick persons who take advantage of humanitarian legislation." [22] Representative Frank Thompson of New Jersey said that if physicians write the nation's laws, he would "have a hand at writing out prescriptions." [23] The Trenton *Trentonian* said that it was unthinkable that physicians as a group would revolt against a law of the land, but that the resolution created the impression in the public mind that the Point Pleasant physicians would go so far as to deny medical care to the aged. It said that of course there was no such intent because even the physicians signing the resolution said that they would treat the indigent elderly without charge, if necessary. The *Trentonian* remarked that even in view of these statements by the physicians the reaction became so strong that extreme measures were suggested, typified by a bill introduced in the state legislature "providing for loss of license, a jail sentence and a fine for rebellious physicians." [24]

The bill to punish "rebellious physicians" so enraged the president of the Medical Society of New Jersey, Ralph M. L. Buchanan, that he issued a statement published in New Brunswick as an advertisement at the expense of the Middlesex County Medical Society, and also published elsewhere throughout the state.[25] Dr. Buchanan admitted that he had not seen the bill, but said: "I find it difficult to believe that any duly constituted public legislative body of the United States of America would so far disregard the fundamental guarantees of liberty and justice for all as seriously to consider for passage a piece of legislation such as this is reported to be. This is a legislative proposal that belongs in a police state. There is no question here of violation of an anachronistic oath taken to some false pagan gods. This bill violates and outrages the Constitution of the United States and imperils the basic rights of every citizen." Speaking of the freedom of the physician and of the patient, he writes, "the physician engages, on the basis of terms agreed upon, to render a service. The patient accepts the terms for that service, and a mutually binding contract is freely entered into. Freedom is essential to the validity of that contract. Even labor leaders should understand that."

Dr. Buchanan certainly recognized the emotionalism inherent in the proposed plan to punish physicians, but he contradicted centuries of experience when he attempted to deny all humanitarianism within the practice of medicine and place it strictly upon a contractual, business-is-business relationship. Obviously, the physician has responsibilities that do not affect the ordinary business arrangement, but just as obviously the patient cannot, because of this, be given an unlimited claim upon all services of the physician. Both the original Point Pleasant "manifesto" and the bill to punish recalcitrant physicians reflect the prevailing emotionalism engendered by the health insurance issue and illustrate the violence of the controversy.

One of the most interesting features of the campaign for and against the Anderson-King Bill was a phonograph recording, "Ronald Reagan Speaks Out Against Socialized Medicine." Mr. Reagan, then a motion picture actor, was just beginning his active career in politics that has carried him to the governorship of California and prominence in the national circles of the Republican Party. The recording was the heart of the American Medical Association's "Operation Coffeecup" to encourage supporters of the position taken by organized medicine to write to their senators and representatives. The recording was strictly for limited circulation and was not designed to win support from those not already committed.

The Woman's Auxiliary to the American Medical Association conducted Operation Coffeecup at the request of its parent organization. The auxiliary distributed the recording to its members accompanied by a letter on its official stationery. The jacket of the recording included detailed instructions as to its use for maximum effect in eliciting letters to members of Congress. The text of the letter stressed the importance of the project to each member, and to American medicine in its efforts to combat "socialized medicine." The member was to list the number of times played, the size of the audience, and the number of letters sent to Congress, along with her own name, address, and auxiliary on the report form. The form provided spaces for listing one through six playings.

The text on the jacket begins by stating the problem: "The legislative chips are down. In the next few months Americans will decide whether or not this nation wants socialized medicine. . . . Proponents admit the bill is a 'foot in the door' for socialized medicine. Its eventual effect—across-the-board, government medicine for everyone"! It explains that "film star Ronald Reagan effectively expresses his own views about the dangers of government in medicine. This new, thought-provoking record is the property of the Woman's Auxiliary. It can be the instrument for eliciting thousands of letters opposing the King bill and similar legislation."

The Association's publicity experts carefully designed the instructions for conducting "Operation Coffeecup." The auxiliary members were instructed to listen to the recording, read the literature accompanying it to "learn as much as you can about the King bill and why it is 'bad medicine' "; then, to "put on the coffeepot," invite friends and neighbors in for coffee, and play the record for them. The members were asked to read the leaflet "Medical Aid for the Aged," to "draw information to state the case against legislation like the King bill," before their friends arrived. According to the instructions, it was important to discuss the issue thoroughly after playing the recording, because the friends would "raise questions you'll have to answer." The members also were directed to stress to their visitors that Mr. Reagan had made the recording from conviction and had received no pay for it.

After the discussion "should come action—in the form of let-

ters from your guests to congressmen in your district and senators in your state. These letters should express personal opposition to socialized medicine in general and to the King bill
(H.R. 4222) in particular." The auxiliary members were not to
miss any opportunity that might result in a letter. "Make letter-
writing easy" say the instructions; "provide each guest with
stationery, pens and stamped envelopes. Don't accept an 'I'll do
it tomorrow' reply—urge each woman to write her letters while
she's in your house—and in the mood! Advise your guests that
letters should be short and to the point, objecting to the King
bill (H.R. 4222) and giving reasons for opposing it. Each woman should write her own letter in her own words, not merely
copy a stereotyped form. See that each woman addresses her
own letters to her own congressmen on the spot. You can mail
them all later. A list of congressmen, with instructions for addressing letters to them, is enclosed."

After repeating the sessions until all possibilities were exhausted, the member was instructed to pass the material along
to other Auxiliary members and was reminded that every mo-
ment counted. The instructions included a list of ten suggestions
from the U. S. Chamber of Commerce regarding effective letters
to members of Congress. These call for proper form, local emphases, individual letterheads and styles, requests for action,
requests for direct answers, appreciation for "good votes" and
for his "better speeches," and praise for his staff.

The instructions include one note of caution regarding the
material: "Remember—this record is especially created for playing to informal groups in homes of individual Auxiliary members." The instructions on the jacket bear the imprint of the
American Medical Association, Communications Division, 535
North Dearborn Street, Chicago 10, Illinois.

The recording is divided into two sections, the first, slightly
over half its length, is a plea by Mr. Reagan for the nation to
halt "socialistic trends"; the second is an unidentified voice that
repeats Reagan's arguments and elaborates upon them, purporting to give some historical background on "socialized medi-

cine." Though the text is a striking exercise in emotionalism, it does not equal the emotional intensity of Mr. Reagan's delivery.

Reagan begins with the apology that it must seem presumptuous for one of his calling to address "anyone on serious problems of the nation and the world. It would be strange," he says, "if it were otherwise." After some brief persiflage, he begins his serious task with quotations purportedly from former Socialist leader Norman Thomas, to the effect that "liberalism" will result in "socialism." He follows with the statement that "there are many ways in which our government has invaded the precincts of private citizens, the method of earning a living," and that the government now owns "a fifth of the total industrial capacity of the United States."

After the brief introduction and general material, he begins his attack upon the health care program. "One of the traditional methods of imposing statism or socialism on a people," he says, "has been by way of medicine. It's very easy to disguise a medical program as a humanitarian project." Since the American people would "unhesitatingly" reject socialized medicine "if you put it to them," as was done, he says, under the Truman Administration, it was necessary for its sponsors to present the program little by little, subscribing to a "foot in the door philosophy." He quotes Walter Reuther to the effect that the United Automobile Workers Union backs a program of national health insurance, and says that "by national health insurance he meant socialized medicine for every American."

Reagan proceeds to charge the bill's sponsors with emotionalism, to quote James Madison, and, by implication, to criticize the social security program itself. He agrees that "very few of us" would criticize the "original premise that there should be some form of saving that would keep destitution from following unemployment by reason of death, disability, or old age, and to this end social security was adopted. But it was never intended to supplant private savings, private insurance, pension programs of unions and industries." He cites freedom of choice of physicians and says that the people must protect it and the freedom of the physician to practice. "A doctor would be reluctant to say this," he says. "Well, like you, I'm only a patient so I can say it in his behalf." He speaks of the freedom the physician "loses" under the bill and wonders whether anyone has the right so to abridge the freedom of another human being. "I know how I'd feel if you my fellow citizens, decided that to be an actor I had to become a government employee and work in a national theater."

He praises the Founding Fathers and the American Revolution, but says that today we "talk democracy . . . and, strangely, we let democracy begin to assume the aspect of majority rule is all that is needed." To protect the rights of the minority, he calls for letters to Washington and points out that this is not the same as writing fan mail to a television program. He says that only "40,000 letters, less than 100 per congressman, are evidence of a trend in public thinking." Then he gives instructions for proper addressing, adding:

> . . . if this man writes back to you and tells you that he, too, is for free enterprise, but we must have these great services, and so forth that must be performed by government, don't let him get away with it. Show that you have not been convinced. Write a letter right back and tell him that you believe in government economy and fiscal responsibility, that you know that governments don't tax to get the money they need, governments will always find a need for the money they get, and that you demand the continuation of our traditional free enterprise system. You and I can do this. The only way we can do it is by writing to our congressman, even if we believe that he's on our side to begin with. Write to strengthen his hand. Give him the ability to stand before his colleagues in Congress and say, I heard from my constituents and this is what they want. Write those letters now; call your friends and tell them to write them. If you don't, this program, I promise you, will pass just as surely as the sun will come up tomorrow. And behind it will come other federal programs that will invade every area of freedom as we have known it in this country. Until one day, as Norman Thomas said, we will awake

to find that we have socialism. And if you don't do this and if
I don't do it, one of these days you and I are going to spend our
sunset years telling our children and our children's children
what it once was like in America when men were free.

As Reagan's voice fades away, that of the announcer enters
to give some background on "socialized medicine, which simply
means compulsory national health insurance; medicine controlled and administered by the federal government financed
through compulsory taxation." Surveys "prove," he says, that
most of the aged are in "reasonably good health" and "reasonably good shape financially." The Kerr-Mills Law permits the
states to guarantee the health care he requires "to every American over 65," and the Anderson-King Bill would be limited in
benefits. After explaining that social security taxes would be
used to pay the expenses, he says, "I am sure many of you are
wondering why there is any objection to using the Social Security System to finance medical care for the aged. Well, first of all,
it is a misnomer to think of Social Security as being insurance."

In substance, in addition to cost and some predictions concerning other programs that would restrict American freedom,
the basic argument of the announcer is that the word "insurance" when applied to social security is inaccurate, and that
the program is therefore unsound. Though the text of the recording seems extreme, it is characteristic of the campaign
against the Administration's health care program. The AMA
and its allied organizations have used all the charges hurled by
Reagan and the announcer. Many were also brought into the
1961 Ways and Means Committee hearings and into the subsequent debates in both Houses of Congress, and they were used
continually until the passage of Medicare in 1965.

Such efforts were intensified by the activities of AMPAC, the
American Medical Political Action Committee, formed on the
pattern of organized labor's Committee on Political Education
to spearhead the political fight. One of the association's major
intents, as illustrated by the Reagan recording, was to encour-

age letters to Congress. Other activities included attempts to defeat proponents of health-care legislation, making use of car pools to transport voters to the polls, and frequent speeches to civic groups. The threat of the Anderson-King Bill was the major impetus for the formation of AMPAC; and Dr. Annis, then head of the AMA's speakers bureau, remarked, "like it or not ... the physician must acknowledge that his profession has been thrown, willynilly, into the political arena." The AMA Board of Trustees selects the ten AMPAC directors, and the AMA supports it financially, but AMPAC's greatest financial support comes from contributions, including those from the executives of drug companies. Despite secrecy regarding its membership, financial, and organizational details, it is known that it operates through local committees in every jurisdiction.[26]

During the stormy controversy of 1962, charges, counter-charges, and threats flew back and forth at a rapid and confusing rate. The New Jersey boycott plan brought similar talk from other medical groups throughout the country. Dr. Annis frequently asserted that the bill would be a bonanza for the rich, and a "cruel hoax" for the poor. In March the Democratic National Chairman, John M. Bailey, charged in a Denver speech that the AMA was becoming an "ally of the John Birch Society in a surgical mask," and that the "self-perpetuating, bureaucratic dynasty that controls the AMA has stood for years against the social and economic advances that the Birch Society stands against today." In May, the Administration scheduled numerous rallies throughout the nation to hear top government speakers advance the cause of the bill. Not only were top Administration figures employed, but several high-ranking civil servants from within the Social Security Administration as well. This caused many of these men a good deal of apprehension, though they firmly supported the bill personally, because they feared reprisals from opponents based upon allegations that they may have violated the Hatch Act that forbids civil servants from taking part in politics. Fortunately for the men involved there were no questions regarding their roles; but the Hatch

Act reinforces, quite understandably, the timidity that exists within the top reaches of this agency.

There were questions, however, regarding the rallies. The AMA's president Dr. Larson charged that they constituted a "massive propaganda blitz designed to pressure Congress." He said that the Treasury was being "looted to help subsidize the biggest lobbying campaign this nation has ever seen." "How," he asked, "were the rallies organized? Who is masterminding and coordinating them? Who is really behind the National Council of Senior Citizens? Where is this organization getting its money and why isn't it registered as a lobbyist?" He mentioned that "hordes" of government employees and federal officials were roaming throughout the country at government expense, and that this was a flagrant violation of the law prohibiting the use of federal employees for lobbying.

In a similar attack, Dr. Blasingame protested that the Department of Health, Education, and Welfare had released propaganda material directly in support of the proposed bill, and he called for a congressional investigation. The booklet in question, the Department's *The Health Care of the Aged,* was a summary of the health needs and the financial condition of the aged, and strongly asserted the need for a health program under the social security system. Dr. Blasingame charged that the publication of the booklet was a criminal act punishable by fine or imprisonment or both, and removal from office, since federal funds were used without direct congressional authorization. Secretary Ribicoff replied that the Justice Department, after an "initial review of the contents of the booklet," suggested that the law had not been violated, and had so notified the AMA by telegram. The Secretary pointed out that HEW has a specific duty, imposed by Congress, to "make recommendations as to the most effective method of providing economic security through social security" and that the publication of the booklet was consistent with its responsibilities. In an apparent attempt to have the last word, the Secretary commented that the charge was an AMA smokescreen to divert attention from the Point

Pleasant situation, but Dr. Annis defended the New Jersey physicians, and said that their motives had been overlooked in "the battle for headlines."

The AMA had also responded vigorously to a comment by President Kennedy during a news conference on May 23 that it had been one of the chief opponents of social security during the 1930's. AMA president Larson said that the allegation was "entirely incorrect," that the AMA had never officially taken a position on the legislation. President Kennedy asked why, if this were true, the December 1939 issue of the *JAMA* had printed the following statement by Dr. Fishbein: "Indeed, all forms of security, compulsory security, even against old age and unemployment, represent a beginning invasion by the state into the personal life of the individual, represent a taking away of individual responsibility, a weakening of national caliber, a definite step toward either communism or totalitarianism." It should be noted here that the AMA's position is that neither *JAMA* editorials nor statements by its president or other officials necessarily represent its official policy, which is embodied solely in resolutions passed by its House of Delegates. It should also be noted that, during its official testimony regarding the passage of the Social Security Act, the AMA did, indeed, take no position. To bolster his charges President Kennedy asked the Association why, if it has not opposed social security, the House of Delegates in 1949 adopted the following resolution: "So-called 'Social Security' is in fact a compulsory socialistic tax which has not provided satisfactory insurance protection for individuals where it has been tried but, instead, has served as the entering wedge for establishment of a socialistic form of government control over the lives and fortunes of the people." To this the AMA merely reiterated its former statement.

The controversy spilled over onto the floor of the House of Representatives when Representative John Dingell (D-Mich.) called Representative Durward Hall (R-Mo.), himself a physician, a mouthpiece for the AMA. Representative Thomas Curtis (R-Mo.) was quick to rise to Representative Hall's defense, and to invoke the House rule barring personal insult. This small issue was settled, however, when Representative Dingell changed "mouthpiece" to "self-appointed spokesman," and Representative Curtis withdrew his objection. Throughout the controversy, Dr. Annis objected to the portrait of the AMA as a "creaking bastion of conservatism" with its "collective heads buried in the sands of time," saying that the conception is amusing but far from the truth. He pointed out that the AMA had not confined its activities to opposition and negativism, but had supported many constructive measures and based its opposition to Medicare on its honest belief that it would result in inferior medicine.

The defeat of the Anderson-Javits amendment in July 1962 was a climactic development in the long and bitter battle. The controversy continued until the final passage of Medicare in 1965, but never at such a fevered pitch as it had attained in 1962, though there are interesting aspects of the later stages of the battle that are considered in some detail below.

ADVERTISING

Following its long-established custom whenever the issue of health care began to dominate the news, the AMA announced on August 17, 1964, that it was embarking upon a major advertising campaign presenting anti-Medicare views. The campaign was to center upon television announcements and would have as its major theme the health care of the aged. The estimated cost of the effort was projected by trade sources to be about one million dollars. AMA plans were dealt a blow, however, when the networks in early September declined to sell time for spot ads. The AMA had sought a series of one-minute periods for dramatized messages, plus one half-hour program for a general discussion. A.E. Duram of the Chicago office of Fuller, Smith, and Ross, Inc., the agency handling the campaign, said that A.B.C. and N.B.C. offered to reconsider if the copy were revised, but that C.B.S. had made a flat refusal.

On September 8, the AMA's executive vice-president, Dr. Blasingame, blasted the networks with the charge of censorship. He said that they were evidently willing to sell one-minute spots to promote the program but not to attack it. Moreover, he denied that the AMA's effort was to be propaganda. He said that it was to have been purely an educational program and not intended to influence legislation because it was not scheduled to have begun until October, by which time the Congress would have "disposed of medicare legislation and adjourned." The AMA merely desired educational time, he said, because most people seemed to be unaware of existing programs that could meet the health-care needs.

The networks responded by denying that they had sold time to promote the program. They said that, with the exception of appearances by political candidates, it was their general policy to confine presentation of controversial subjects to established discussion programs. They believed one minute to be inadequate to present a reasoned examination of an issue. The next day Dr. Blasingame announced that the AMA had received many offers from local stations for time to present its spot ads.

On September 17, the AMA attempted another approach. It demanded equal time on N.B.C.'s "Today" show to answer what it called a "scurrilous attack" on the organization and its former president, Dr. Annis, by Senator Clinton P. Anderson (D-N.M.) who had appeared on the show. Anderson, the Senate sponsor of the Anderson-King proposal, had remarked that the AMA was conducting a propaganda campaign against his bill for which physicians were being asked to contribute $100.00 apiece. The AMA strenuously denied this. The Association did not win equal time, but it won a victory in its contest with the networks when A.B.C. agreed on September 23 to show its one-minute spot ads. Dr. Blasingame said that the network had reconsidered when the AMA had made revisions in the texts to be used. About 150 A.B.C. affiliates and over 140 other stations, primarily in metropolitan areas, carried the announcements.

In another victory, the AMA succeeded in obtaining time from C.B.S. to present its half-hour program on October 18. The network agreed to provide the time without charge, and to provide similar time to the National Council of Senior Citizens on October 25. The AMA program was called "Your Doctor Reports—Again" and it consisted of a discussion of the association's views on health care by Dr. Annis and newsman Bob Considine, who was associated with Mutual of Omaha, one of the leading health insurance companies. The program was related to "Community Health Week," the week from October 18 to 24. Accompanying the telecast effort was a kit of publicity materials sent to the state and local medical societies. Included in the kit was a recommended "ministerial announcement." "It would be well that during this Community Health Week we join in prayer," said the announcement, "in appreciation of the health services provided by the dedicated teams of physicians, nurses, technologists, and all workers who serve our community."

In its last effort to obtain support for its "Eldercare" plan, the AMA announced in early February of 1965 that it was planning to spend over one half million dollars on radio and television spot announcements on the Mutual Broadcasting System and A.B.C. to be heard over hundreds of radio and television stations nationally. One week later it announced that its public relations office was engaged in mailing some seven million pamphlets promoting Eldercare, and attacking Medicare. Included was a reprint of a *Reader's Digest* article by Walter Judd, "Medicare—or Medical Care? We Must Not Play Politics with the Health of the Nation." Again, as so often before, articles from this magazine played a major part in the effort to defeat the health program. Local and state medical societies, and interested groups within the field of medicine and outside it as well, were encouraged to supplement the national AMA effort by campaigns at the local and regional levels.

On June 8, the Chicago office announced that one hundred newspapers throughout the country would carry an advertisement that would make the AMA's position on medicare "clear." The advertisement was headed "Health Care at the Crossroads: An Open Letter to Our Patients." It was signed by AMA president Donovan Ward and continued the themes used throughout previous AMA advertising campaigns, such as claiming that Medicare would be "the beginning of socialized medicine" and urging voters to write critical letters to Congress.[27] The advertisement was keyed to an AMA television program on A.B.C., also titled "Health Care at the Crossroads," on which Dr. Ward and Dr. Annis appeared June 17.

In what it surely considered as one last insult, the AMA discovered that the National Council of Senior Citizens, after having claimed poverty, had received free time from A.B.C. to answer its "Crossroads" program, a program for which the AMA had purchased time. In a tired and angry release, Dr. Blasingame charged that the National Council was nothing more than a "lobbying appendage" for the labor unions and the Democratic National Committee. In utter disregard of this charge, the National Council's program featured, among others, Nelson Cruikshank, director of social security for the AFL-CIO, Commissioner Robert M. Ball of the Social Security Administration, and Vice President Hubert H. Humphrey.

THE AMA AND MR. NORMILE

Soon after its formation, the political-action arm of organized medicine, AMPAC, threw itself into its task with gusto, as has been noted earlier. AMPAC's zeal was so great that when it was hardly more than a year old, it caused the AMA one of the most embarrassing incidents in the history of the venerable organization and brought it face-to-face with a $400,000 suit for damages resulting from alleged fraud and libel. In November of 1963, Mr. Paul Normile, director of the western Pennsylvania district 16 of the United Steelworkers of America, filed the suit against the AMA in Federal Court in Washington, D.C.

The suit stemmed from a phonograph recording that the AMA produced in quantity and distributed by the thousands throughout the country. The recording purported to be of a speech by Normile at a political education meeting of a group of steelworkers in western Pennsylvania. The voice on the recording made rough threats in gangsterlike fashion as though extorting contributions from assembled union members to support the battle for medicare by threatening those who did not "come across" with the "graveyard shift" and other unpleasantness. The voice was tough-talking and at least semi-illiterate.

The president of the AFL-CIO, George Meany, asserted that the recording was an "absolute fraud." Normile denied that the recorded voice was his or that he had made any such speech. Meany denied that any such speech had been made by anyone. The record jacket, entitled the "Voice of COPE," contained a printed text of the recording and information to the effect that AMPAC had obtained it from a union member, one "who opposes, as many members of the labor movement do, the high-pressure methods which C.O.P.E. resorts to in its efforts to dominate government at every level within the United States." A message on the jacket, signed by Donald E. Wood, M.D., chairman of the board of directors of AMPAC, recommended that the record be played to make physicians aware that membership in AMPAC is essential for the maintenance of free medical practice. The AMA decided to withhold official comment on the suit until it became aware of the full details, but Dr. Annis called the charges "ridiculous" and merely an effort to divert attention from the issues.

The following January the judge rejected a plea by the union that the AMA be ordered to apologize in the *JAMA* for having distributed the record. The judge ruled that this would be an admission of guilt. The court proceedings reveal that the record was purchased for twenty dollars on a dark street late at night from an unknown middleman. The AMA represented the suit as actually a dispute between organized medicine and organized labor regarding pending legislation. For a time, its spokesman maintained that it was merely an effort to discredit the association and said that they had not eliminated the possibility that the voice actually did belong to Normile, even though a speech expert that Normile hired had asserted that it was not possible. They admitted that the AMA did not know whose voice was on the recording but that it had been thought to be authentic when purchased. They further maintained that it was the privilege of the association to distribute the recording because it dealt with pending legislation of great importance and national interest and that the association should not, therefore, be held liable for damages. The judge refused to permit the record to be played in court, but he listened to a transcript read by the attorney for Normile and the union.

After a long delay and much bargaining and hesitation the AMA announced on March 11, 1966, that it had arrived at a settlement out of court with Mr. Normile, and issued a statement that was printed in the following issue of the *JAMA* and carried on page one of the *AFL-CIO News* for March 12:

In March 1963, the Ameircan Medical Association was sent a tape recording of what purported to be a political fund raising speech made in Pennsylvania by a Pittsburgh labor leader, Mr. Paul Normile, director of District 16, United Steelworkers of America. Believing in good faith that the tape recording was authentic, the AMA reproduced it and the American Medical Political Action Committee produced and distributed a booklet entitled 'The Voice of COPE', containing the text of the speech and a phonograph record made from the tape as evidence of the tactics which they believed labor used in support of its objectives.

Mr. Normile thereafter filed a lawsuit alleging that he never made the speech in question. Distribution of the tapes and records was immediately voluntarily discontinued pending full investigation of his contention. As result of its exhaustive investigation, the AMA is now satisfied that Mr. Normile did not make the speech in question. In fairness to him, the statement that he did so is retracted. Furthermore, all copies of the tape recording and the AMPAC booklet and record in the possession of AMA or AMPAC have been destroyed. To prevent further playing of the recording, it is urged that any person having a copy of either the tape or the record take similar action. The AMA sincerely regrets the error.

The financial settlement was reported to be $25,000. The hesitancy that caused the AMA to wait for two and one half years is understandable. No professional association could admit involvement in such an affair without, at best, a considerable impairment of its dignity.

THE BATTLE FOR ELDERCARE

In January 1965, the AMA moved to kill Medicare by substituting the "Eldercare" proposal. It announced a new "national educational campaign" designed to foster support for what the organization called the "doctors' Eldercare program" and held an emergency meeting of the House of Delegates in Chicago in February to build enthusiasm. The trustees, who had planned and announced the proposal, faced some opposition regarding their request for authorization to spend an unspecified amount from the AMA's reserve fund. The fund was said to contain between four and seven million dollars. The response of the trustees was that organized medicine was in a fight for its very existence, and that the cost could not be estimated. On February 7, the House of Delegates adopted a resolution supporting Eldercare enthusiastically, and reaffirmed the AMA's opposition to the pending legislation.

The substance of the AMA's campaign was that Eldercare would supply more benefits than Medicare and at less cost. An advertisement read: "Your doctors, who care for the elderly, support Eldercare because it also assures free choice of physician and hospital." There were many critics of the plan, however, including some from within the ranks of the AMA. They said that insurance companies could not function under the plan in the absence of national standards. The executive council of the AFL-CIO adopted a formal policy statement at their Bal Harbour, Florida, meeting on February 23 condemning Eldercare and repeating their support of Medicare. The statement accused the AMA's plan of being unworkable and containing "empty promises." Since the states would define the scope of the program within their borders, available benefits would be limited, said the statement, by the amount of state funds on hand to match federal grants. The council said that organized medicine would have the people believe that the trouble with the Anderson-King approach was that it promised too little, yet they recommended the substitution of a "pie-in-the-sky" plan that would merely "authorize" a vast range of benefits in place of the basic hospital insurance that the Medicare bill would actually provide. Though the benefits would be "authorized," said the council, their actual realization would depend on the appropriations of great sums by both Congress and the various state legislatures.

The AMA, fighting a last-ditch battle, needed all the support that it could get, but on March 16 one of its strong supporters added his voice to the chorus of critics. Representative Herlong, who had introduced the Eldercare plan into the House of Representatives, accused the AMA of issuing misleading information in its support. Representative Herlong said that he still supported Eldercare, but that the AMA had attempted to "oversell" it to Congress and to the public and he did not believe this to be in order. He charged that AMA advertising distorted the extent of coverage available under Eldercare. In noting that the advertisements say that Eldercare would provide much broader coverage than Medicare, Mr. Herlong said, "for them to give the impression it provides complete coverage is not so. . . . It just makes it available for the states to provide it if they want to." He said that the advertisements said that Eldercare would provide "complete coverage for those who needed aid" and "100 percent of all expenses. You know and I know that it doesn't do all those things," he added; "it is misleading." Subsequently he issued a second statement to the effect that the Administration's supporters had also exaggerated, but the damage had been done.

When the House approved the Medicare bill on April 8, ignoring the Eldercare substitute, the AMA issued a critical statement. It said that it was unfortunate that the people had been denied the opportunity to learn how the bill would affect their lives and charged that the development of the measure and its House passage had been characterized by "unrestrained haste." "We believe," said the AMA, "in helping the elderly who need help through a program, such as Eldercare, which is administered by the states, not controlled from Washington." People failed to understand the issues, complained the association, saying that the heart of its opposition was directed toward taxing all for the benefit of those past the age of sixty-five who need no help.

The last push for Eldercare came during the Senate hearings. Dr. Ward, the AMA president, criticized the Medicare program as one leading to overuse of the physician's time, and mentioned the difficulty in reducing a program that had once been put into effect. He called, instead, for the Senate to substitute the AMA's Eldercare plan. Senators Anderson and Vance Hartke (D-Ind.) responded that Eldercare would be nothing more than an expansion of the Kerr-Mills program which, they said, had been completely inadequate except in a few states. Dr. Ward responded that Kerr-Mills could easily be expanded, and that it would have been, had not the Department of Health, Education, and Welfare hampered its growth. As noted earlier, the Department denied that it has hampered the development of Kerr-Mills programs in any way. Dr. Ward also asked that the proposed bill eliminate the contemplated coverage of self-employed physicians under social security (OASDI) He ended his testimony with a blast at the American Hospital Association for allegedly leading a drive to make hospitals, as opposed to physicians' offices, the centers of medical care in the United States. Thus, with one last ill-tempered attack upon one of its closest professional allies, the AMA turned to face the defeat of its Eldercare program and, much worse from its point of view, the adoption of legislation establishing health coverage through the social security mechanism.

BOYCOTT THREATS

There had been talk of a boycott by physicians in the event that Congress adopted Medicare since the incident in 1962 at Point Pleasant, New Jersey. As the Medicare thrust gained irresistible momentum in 1965, the talk increased. Several physicians in various portions of the nation assumed leadership of actual boycott movements. On May 12 the Ohio Medical Association voted 77 to 71 to urge physicians to refuse to accept fees from the program on behalf of the patients that they treat. A leader in the Ohio boycott movement, Dr. Jack Schreiber of Canfield, predicted a general boycott. Spokesmen for the Chicago office of the AMA said that they assumed that there would be an effort during the June session of the House of Delegates to make Ohio's policy the national policy of organized medicine. Dr. Ward commented that he did not "like to see this" because he did not wish to give the impression that physicians would neglect patients, even though nothing in the law required them to accept anyone for treatment. Dr. Schreiber had said that he had already informed his patients that he would refuse federal fees directly *or indirectly,* and had received a "fine response." He was one of three physicians in Canfield. The Arizona Medical Association adopted a similar stand.

In May, however, Dr. Ward said that the boycott moves were "untimely and premature" since there had as yet been no action by the Senate, and he urged physicians not to approve them. Dr. Ward was speaking in Tulsa in opposition to a proposed boycott resolution under consideration by the House of Delegates of the Oklahoma State Medical Association. The president of the Oklahoma group, Dr. Harlan Thomas, agreed with Dr. Ward. Ward noted that he considered it "good strategy" not to permit anyone to know what would take place should Medicare be adopted. On May 14, the same day as Ward's speech, the Board of Directors of the San Francisco Medical Society voted unanimously to participate willingly in the governmental program. The Board said that it based its action on reports of threatened "doctors strikes" from various sections of the nation. Similarly, on May 19, the House of Delegates of the Minnesota State Medical Association voted not to boycott the program if it should be enacted. Additional voices opposing a boycott came from New York. On May 24, Dr. John M. Cotton, the outgoing president of the New York County Medical Society, urged other societies to help the new program work, saying that much more was to be gained by cooperation than by obstruction. On May 29, the New York Academy of Medicine, a non-profit association of some two thousand physicians, repudiated the AMA position regarding Medicare and issued a statement saying that health care should be based solely upon health considerations, not economics. It rejected the notion that governmental funds should be administered by private organizations, saying that only a governmental agency combines the necessary authority, skill, and accountability.

But the boycott movements continued. In June, the Association of American Physicians and Surgeons, Inc., sent a notice to virtually every physician in the country urging a boycott of the Medicare program when it began operation. This 15,000-member group is not related to the AMA, and confines its concern to the social and economic aspects of medical practice. The notice was signed by its president, a Ft. Worth, Texas, physician, E. E. Anthony.

When the June meeting of the House of Delegates opened, the greatest support for a boycott came from delegations representing the states of Arizona, Florida, Louisiana, Ohio, Oklahoma, South Carolina, and Texas. The newly-installed president, Dr. James Z. Appel, warned the delegates not to affirm a general boycott movement since such action would be not only unethical but bad citizenship. He requested physicians to co-operate with the "letter and intent of the law," saying that they must be in a position to participate in the development of rules and regulations. He said that "doctors must never let 'political philosophy' influence the care they give patients."

Only a few of the many speakers supported Appel's position. He was loudly accused of "surrender" and "appeasement." Dr. Henriksen, of Point Pleasant fame, was reported as remarking that "force must be used when reason will not prevail." Dr. Annis cautioned the delegates to wait until passage of the bill before action on boycott resolutions since such action might be used against the AMA. Dr. Appel said that he would support whatever the House of Delegates, in its wisdom, should decide. This did not halt a strong feeling of resentment against him from many delegates. On June 24, the House of Delegates rejected calls for a formal boycott but also refused to request physicians to participate. The action left each physician free to participate or not as he saw fit.

The controversy did not subside. In July, the St. Louis Coun-ty Medical Society issued a statement called (with unconscious irony) the "Patient's Bill of Rights," urging a boycott. The statement was adopted in a private meeting of two hundred physicians. In New Jersey, Dr. Henriksen again spoke out pub-licly, saying that under no circumstances would he treat pa-tients under Medicare, and that if it became necessary he would limit his practice to those under the age of sixty-five. The Chi-cago office of the AMA nevertheless tempered the zeal of the boycott leaders somewhat when it warned physicians on August 11 that a concerted boycott could expose them to antitrust ac-tion. It was careful to mention that individual physicians could still boycott the program but cautioned them against organized action. Six days later Dr. Appel announced that he expected many physicians to refuse to participate. He said that he had heard of no one who would refuse patients (apparently he had not heard of Dr. Henriksen's statement) but that many on an individual basis would refuse to complete the necessary government forms that would be required to receive payment.

NOTES ON THE ROLE OF ORGANIZED MEDICARE

True to its traditions, organized medicine attacked the Medicare proposal with a vigor certainly unmatched in the history of American professional organizations, and hardly equalled anywhere on the American scene. It persisted in its strenuous opposition until long after passage of the plan was a foregone conclusion. The intensity of its opposition to health care measures of the last two decades or so has been such that many of its critics have been blinded to the solid accomplishments of the association, and the association itself seems at times to have placed other considerations ahead of its professional programs. The election of Dr. Annis as AMA president suggests that professional matters may not have been uppermost in the minds of the delegates at the 1962 House of Delegates meeting, and connection with such episodes as the fraudulent phonograph recording purporting to be the voice of a union leader can only reflect discredit upon the organization.

Countless episodes of professional boycotts of individual physicians by local medical societies for other than professional reasons have been amply documented. Similar boycotts have been directed at non-physicians. In September 1964, Senator Birch Bayh (D-Ind.) was forced to cancel a "non-political" Medicare speech before a group of pharmacists in Ft. Wayne, Indiana, because they allegedly had been warned to stay away or face loss of business, if they owned pharmacies, or loss of employment if not self-employed. These activities certainly may not be characteristic of organized medicine in general but they have recurred with disturbing frequency and are probably responsible for some of the more extreme charges by anti-AMA critics. Representative Frank Thompson, Jr. (D-N.J.), for example, when the AMA supported the position of the tobacco industry with regard to the labelling of cigarette packages with a health warning, suggested that it had done so in violation of the principles of good health in order to obtain support from the industry against Medicare. The AMA called the charge ridiculous and said that it was utterly without foundation. Whatever the truth of such allegations, the fact that they could even be considered suggests that the violence of the controversy has produced an unhealthy situation, and that the political activities that have catapulted the AMA into the forefront of lobbying organizations make strange bedfellows with medicine's stated professional principles.

The closing note, with a strangely ironic twist, comes from the man who for years represented the AMA to the public, Morris Fishbein, M. D. Dr. Fishbein not only authored the official history of the AMA, but during his long editorship of the *JAMA* became identified, as much as any other single person, with the most extreme of AMA positions regarding the role of government in the health field. He often expressed his view of such involvement with recourse to characteristically colorful terms such as "medical soviets" and "peasant medicine." In June 1965, however, he observed that the AMA could have increased its influence on legislation and governmental health care considerably had it worked to help develop and shape the programs, rather than insisting upon complete acceptance of its negative position. He noted that the American Hospital Association had followed the more moderate and cooperative course and had been effective in modifying proposed legislation. He said that the AMA's efforts had ended "on a downbeat" when its president Dr. Ward testified before the Senate Finance Commitee aware that the cause had already been lost. "After nearly two decades of struggle and controversy, million-dollar advertising drives, rallies, and political action campaigns, the AMA's crusade had failed, and in the opinion of many knowledgeable people in Washington, the AMA's own strategy of uncompromising resistance contributed to the di-

mensions of its defeat." He added that the AMA increased the
irony of the situation by closing its "year of anti-Medicare testimony in Congress with an unusual attack, not on the Johnson
Administration or organized labor, but on the American Hospital Association." He called this a reflection of the "major decline in the AMA's power position, not only in Washington but
in the health field generally." [28]

The irony, of course, was as much in the shift of position by
Dr. Fishbein as it was in the liklihood that the intensive efforts
of the AMA had contributed to its own defeat. Most ironic of
all was the statement that he made in Baltimore on October
29. "As conditions change, we must adapt to the changes. . . .
When conditions become so severe they can no longer be handled by private initiative, the Government must step in." He
now supports federal health programs, including Medicare.[29]

In all probability the passage of the program of health benefits through social security will be beneficial to the professional
activities of the AMA. No longer will organized medicine be
terrified by the spectre of a government program that, if it is
only resisted sufficiently, might be averted. The AMA has a history of opposing new programs, yet accepting them after they
have been established and cooperating fully. Soon after enactment of the program, the association announced that it would
assist the government in setting policy for Medicare, and would
help the program to work in order to escape the blame for any
harmful effects. There is every reason to believe that the possibility of such harmful effects will be greatly lessened by AMA
cooperation.

VI

rhetorical reconciliation in the u. s. senate

The preceding chapters dealing with the general issues of social security and Medicare illustrate forcefully the role of the rhetorical reconciliation in modern society. In order to apply a similar anaylsis to the actual legislative process, this chapter turns to an examination of the most heated of all Congressional Medicare debates—those occurring in the summer of 1962 regarding the proposals of the Kennedy Administration. For purposes of comparison, the Senate debates prior to Medicare's passage in 1965 are also examined.

When it became apparent that the Ways and Means Committee would not report the Anderson-King Bill to the House, Senate sponsors attempted to attach it as an amendment to a House-approved measure, H.R. 10606, the Public Welfare Amendments of 1962. The chances for Senate passage seemed good, but to improve them further the sponsors dropped the original Anderson-King Bill (H. R. 4222 and S. 909) in favor of a compromise, the Anderson-Javits proposal. The bill thus gained an air of bipartism support since five Republicans joined with the twenty-two Democrats as sponsors. In the final vote, however, the five Republican sponsors were the only Republicans opposing the motion to table.

The important compromise provisions were the "blanketing in" of all persons who would reach the age of sixty-five before 1967 without social security coverage (to be financed by funds from the general revenues) ; the use of private organizations to perform certain administrative functions at the request of hospitals or other participating health facilities; and a limited option allowing beneficiaries to continue private health insurance coverage if they wished. This rather complicated option, it should be noted, did not actually provide for government financing of private insurance. Under certain specific conditions a beneficiary who had been covered by an approved plan for five years preceding his retirement could elect to continue such coverage. To be approved, the company or sponsor of the plan had to meet rigid requirements, such as operating nationwide or else receiving a large percentage of the insurance business in areas in which it was in operation, and it had to offer services equivalent to those offered by the federal program *plus* "some additional services." The beneficiary would pay a premium only for the "additional services," and the company would receive no other payment on his behalf unless and until he used some covered health services and requested payment; whereupon the government would reimburse the private company the amount it actually had paid for the services, plus an amount for the company's administrative expenses.[1]

In effect, the beneficiary would have had a small private policy, at his expense, providing benefits beyond those covered by the government, and the carrier would have been a fiscal agent making payments on behalf of the federal program. This is an example of an attempt to rationalize a government program by the adoption of the symbols, mostly rhetorical (for example, "private-insurance option") , of the American ideology.

After extensive debate, the opponents of the amendment moved that it be tabled. With the unexpected support of Senator Jennings Randolph (D-W. Virginia) , a sponsor of the bill, the motion carried and the health plan was defeated for that session of Congress. Senator Randolph subsequently explained that he had voted to table the amendment because of fear that its adoption would delay the passage of the Public Welfare Amendments which he considered vital to his state of West Virginia.[2] As an interesting sidelight upon the unexpected defeat of the proposal, Senator Anderson has charged that Robert G. Baker, the former secretary to the Senate majority who resigned from his post because of questions surrounding his financial dealings, "offered to help" on the health care vote. "Anderson showed Baker his estimate of every Senator's position on the measure. Anderson's list included four Senators he thought would probably vote for the bill and give him a slim majority." Anderson says that Baker's list "agreed with his on all but two Senators against whom question marks were registered." Even without their votes Anderson figured that healthcare would win. He says that he believes Baker "carried this information to Kerr [Sen. Robert Kerr (D-Okla), co-author of the Kerr-Mills Bill]; and, like a dentist probing, Kerr found the cavities and drilled and enlarged them." Anderson has not named the four Senators whom he considered as doubtful, but he has said that none of them supported the bill. Senator Randolph was also concerned about losing a Kerr amendment that cleared away a legal cloud over West Virginia's $11 million in payments to jobless fathers. Passage of this provision enabled the state to continue a welfare program that had been halted.[3]

The Senate debates on the motion to table the Anderson-Javits Amendment are excellent sources for illustrations of certain general tendencies of the culture, and of particular workings of the American political process. Distortions of language are readily evident in the efforts of Senators on both sides of the question to support their positions and achieve a "rhetorical reconciliation" with the demands of the American ideology, on the one hand, or to demonstrate variance from that ideology, on the other. Since the American ideology, following the precedents established during the time of the New Deal, may now be used to support a program of social security incorporating the traditional symbols, the proponents could point to the amendment's consistency with American tradition; similarly, the opponents associated it with foreign programs and a departure from the accepted principles of social security, as well as from the major traditions of the eighteenth and nineteenth centuries. Apart from general references, the proponents specifically emphasized American traditions somewhat more than did opponents. On six occasions, five supporters included "consistency with American traditions" as major portions of their debating efforts. Four opponents, on four occasions, used heavy emphasis upon tradition as a major point.

The following analysis borrows, and modifies, the techniques of "content analysis" to examine the Senate debates on the amendment from the date of its introduction, June 29, 1962, to its final tabling on July 17. As the preceding example indicates, the modifications to the technique are considerable. They eschew the usual "word counts" as being somewhat of an oversimplication. Specific words employed by a speaker are subject to so many influences as to be less reliable as an indication of his actual meaning than the substance of his speech. Moreover, the results of content analysis seem insufficient to serve as sound bases for inference; accordingly, the results here are used merely as illustrations.

This analysis compares the reactions of the supporters of the amendment to those of its opponents. It does not trace the positions of individual senators throughout the debates to compare their reactions, nor is it limited to the counting of specific phrases or the number of times they occur. Rather, it concentrates upon certain major emphases of the opponents and the supporters as groups. There is no attempt to include all major emphases, only those most relevant to this study. For example, the analysis ignores the relative emphases upon the costs of the program though this was one of the foremost points of criticism by the opponents, and similarly one of the features most heavily defended by proponents. In each case, it measures the number of times (separate occasions) that each group emphasized a certain point, as well as the number of senators of each group who emphasized it. Vagaries of phrasing do not affect the outcomes of the analysis. It includes all the material of the debates, colloquiums, statements, and insertions in the *Congressional Record*.

This material occupies almost one-fifth of the total space in the *Record* during the period studied, giving some indication of the importance of the issue. Also valuable as evidence of the degree of interest is the high volume of mail concerning Medicare received by senators.[4]

The analysis supports the thesis that both major parties to public debate in the United States tend to accept certain basic principles and symbols of the American ideology, each side tending to use many of the same symbols to justify positions directly in contradiction to one another. An example of this is the usage of the terms "radical," "liberal," and "conservative." Although most supporters of the amendment would not have hesitated to term themselves "liberals," many of them adopted the term "conservative" to use in praise of the amendment. Only forty-five senators participated in the debates, nineteen opponents and twenty-six supporters. On nine separate occasions, eight of the supporters, almost one-third of those participating, spoke favorably of the plan's "conservatism." The opponents called it "radical" throughout the debates, indicating that "radicalism" as opposed to "conservatism" is undesirable. These eight supporters, ostensibly accepting the same thought, solicited votes for the amendment partially because it was not "radical," because it was sound and conservative." [5]

Similarly, the supporters referred more often to the insurance mechanisms of social security than did opponents. Four opponents on four separate occasions discussed social security as insurance (twice to question whether it is insurance at all) and ten proponents on eleven separate occasions used the insurance-company model of social security to justify their support of the amendment.

A majority of those participating in the debates, both opponents and proponents, based their arguments upon the symbols of private enterprise. The opponents tended to take the position that the "private sector of the economy" was more efficient than the governmental and could perform with greater safeguards to freedom. The supporters tended to praise the bill because of its use of private mechanisms which, they argued, added the advantages of a private program. Thus, at least implicitly, the arguments of both sides paid tribute to private, as opposed to governmental, programs. The frequency for supporters is twenty-eight separate arguments by twelve senators; for opponents, twenty-two arguments by thirteen senators. Additionally, five supporters either discussed the likelihood of beneficial effects on the private insurance industry if the amendment should be passed, or implied that there would be a beneficial effect by pointing to the growth of the industry simultaneously with the growth of social security. Four of these also spoke to the question of the "private sector." Therefore, the combined figures dealing with arguments for private enterprise by supporters of the governmental program are thirty-two separate arguments by thirteen senators.

On the other hand, not all supporters accepted the rhetoric or the desirability of involving private enterprise. Senator Oren E. Long (D-Haw.) said that the government should not use social security funds to "pay profits to private insurance companies" (p. 11874). Senator Pat McNamara (D-Mich.) also criticized the involvement of private organizations (p. 11876). Senator Gale McGee (D-Wyo.) probed to the heart of the issue by remarking with irony that funds to provide for the construction of hospitals were in a different category from those used to pay hospital bills. Support for hospital construction, he said, "is called incentive. That is incentive to a more vigorous private practice of medicine. We cannot call that socialism." His remarks illustrate the flexibility of the notion of private enterprise as well as that of the term "socialism" (p. 12059).

The examination of the use of the word "socialism" provides one of the most interesting sets of figures in the analysis: more supporters based significant portions of their arguments upon the concept of "socialism" than did opponents. Without exception all those employing it as a major debate point condemned it. The disagreement concerned only the character of the amendment, with supporters saying that is was not socialism and opponents saying that it was, or else would be the "entering wedge." Eleven proponents on seventeen occasions argued the point, whereas only nine opponents on thirteen occasions did so. This is a salient example of the acceptance of identical verbal symbols by those on both sides of the argument without regard to relevance.

There were, however, several senators who attempted to inject notes of reason into this segment of the controversy. Senator Wayne Morse (D-Ore.), a strong proponent and one of the sponsors of the amendment, remarked early in the debate that the charge of socialism was an "old bromide" and that he was "not interested in labels" (p. 11436). Senator Jack R. Miller (R-Iowa), an equally strong opponent, likewise said, "Whether the Anderson-Javits program is socialized medicine or is not socialized medicine is not, in my judgment, the question" (p. 12389). Senators Maurine Neuberger (D-Ore.) and McGee in a colloquy agreed that "socialism" was a "scare word" that people should disregard. They proceeded, seemingly with tongue in cheek, to taunt their opponents by saying that the provisions of the Kerr-Mills Act are "close to socialized medicine" (pp. 12058-12059). Senator Stephen Young (D-Ohio), also shrugged off the term as an "AMA scare word" during the course of a trenchant attack upon that organization, which he charged was run by "political doctors" (p. 12626).

There was great variety in the expressions regarding governmental activity. Senator Russell Long (D-La.) went beyond those arguing the question of socialism to say, ". . . it has been my impression that much of the propaganda in behalf of compulsory medical insurance comes alarmingly close to the familiar communist line" (p. 12745). Senator Gordon Allot (R-Colo.) similarly foresaw a plot: "There seems to be a substantial group of people who want to destroy the traditional division of powers, replacing them with centralized concentration of control far removed from the people" (p. 12662). Elsewhere he charged that ". . . this proposal relies on compulsion and denial of freedom, it proclaims the state superior to the individual; it violates Judeo-Christian teachings because it rejects the divinity of man" (p. 12363).

In his praise of the American system of private medical practice, it is noteworthy that Senator Wallace Bennett (R-Utah) pointed with pride to "our medical schools, which are recognized the world over as the best in existence" (p. 12185) but which tend also to be within governmental institutions or within private institutions enjoying heavy governmental subsidies. In contrast, Senator Frank E. Moss (D-Utah) (p. 12654) and New Jersey's Democratic Senator Harrison Williams (p. 12913), echo an argument popular at the time of the passage of the Social Security Act. Essentially, the argument is that a governmental program will prevent other governmental programs from coming into being; the Anderson-Javits Amendment would provide a "bulwark against socialism" or an "antidote to socialism."

The one pertinent subject stressed significantly more by opponents than by supporters was that involving the organization of health care in other countries. It had seemed reasonable to anticipate a result similar to that obtained in examining the use of the concept of socialism; but instead, nine opponents, on eleven separate occasions, made significant reference to the British National Health Service, with the comparable figures for proponents being four senators and seven significant references. For allusions to foreign systems other than that of Great Britain, the disparity is even greater. Not one supporter devoted time to a comparison of the American arrangement with non-British foreign systems, but eight opponents, on ten separate occasions, did so. The closest supporters came to the issue was to argue occasionally, as indicated earlier, that the program was specifically "American," being based upon "American" thought and tradition.

The foreign symbol, therefore, may have been somewhat less

potent to the supporters than to the opponents, although all
those supporters who touched upon it attempted to prove that
the proposed program was uniquely American, hence desirable.
Senator Anderson was the one senator who discussed the British National Health Service without condemnation. Pointing
out that the Administration's health plan was not at all similar
to that existing in Britain (as, indeed, it was not), he said that
much of the criticism in this country of the British system is
unwarranted, and that the extent of American misinformation
about NHS is great. Along with his remarks he included an
article from *The Washington Post* entitled "Britain Likes Its
Medical Program" (pp. 11902-11903).

Two other important emphases in the debates are worth noting, though they are not related specifically to the common acceptance of American ideological symbols by opposing parties
to political debate. One emphasis was that upon parliamentary
procedure, and the other was upon expressions of public opinion measured by private public-opinion polls. The frequency of
references to public-opinion polls and mail from constituents
has not been tabulated, but both sides used them extensively to
support their arguments, with the opponents clearly stressing
them more. Many senators and representatives conducted informal polls of their constituents and reported the results to the
Congress. As could have been expected, most of the polls merely reflect the political coloration of the district that sent the
poll-taker to Congress.

Some members of Congress conduct polls that conform to
rigid standards, but these are few and are limited, of necessity,
to those members possessing independent wealth. Donald R.
Matthews is certainly correct when he says that "most polls by
members of Congress are simply public-relations gimmicks. The
'sampling' is sloppy, the questions loaded, and the data on
public attitudes obtained are of very dubious value." [6] It is
most rare to find one based upon statistical samplings or controlled in any way to eliminate or to reduce bias. They tend
to evidence the same degree of sophistication as Senator Allot's
remark, in reference to a poll of magazine and newspaper edi-

tors showing 78 percent opposed to the Anderson-King Bill and 84 percent favoring a private over a government plan, that "It is reasonable to assume that most of these editors reflect the majority opinion of their readers" (p. 12368).

A major opponent of the Anderson-Javits Amendment, Senator Bennett, inserted a table giving the results of the health-care polls conducted by the members of the Eighty-Seventh Congress, mainly by representatives. The table clearly illustrates the weakness of the polls. Of the fifty-two listed, Democrats conducted only twelve. Of the nineteen favoring the social security mechanism to finance health care, Democrats conducted ten; only two Democratic polls, therefore, rejected the proposal and these were polls by conservative Southern Democrats, one from Texas and one from Arkansas. Only three Southern Democrats were represented in the polls, the third being from Florida, a state that in many respects is politically a border state, and one that in any event is known to attract many retired persons who might be expected to be especially pleased with the prospects of a medicare program.

Considering the character of the polling efforts, the nine Republican polls out of forty that favored the program may even indicate a greater degree of popular support than could have been expected—that is, if there is any value at all other than political to a poll taken under such conditions.

TABLE I

COMPILATION OF POLLS CONDUCTED BY MEMBERS OF CONGRESS

Public opinion on the use of the social security mechanism to finance health care for the aged as tabulated from congressional polls during the 87th Cong.

	For	Against	No opinion
1. Alger (Republican), Texas—5th District, C.R. June 14, 1962, A4427	1,890	25,760	350

2. Ashbrook (Republican), Ohio—17th District, June 12, 1961, A4204	2,019	9,718	883
3. Baldwin (Republican), California—6th District, Mar. 26, 1962, A2281	15,609	6,638	1,752
4. Beall (Republican), Maryland—Senator, May 4, 1962, A3317	355	1,608	290
5. Berry (Republican), South Dakota—2d District, Mar. 15, 1962, A1985	1,024	5,376	....
6. Bolton (Republican), Ohio—22d District, Mar. 5, 1962, A1625	8,295	6,015	690
7. Brademas (Democrat), Indiana—3d District, June 21, 1962, A4707	10,811	7,429	760
8. Bray (Republican), Indiana—7th District, June 13, 1962, A4382	4,200	9,520	280
9. Broyhill (Republican), Virginia—10th District, Mar. 21, 1962, A2180	4,528	10,064	1,408
10. Chamberlain (Republican), Michigan—6th District, Apr. 11, 1962, p. 5916	7,800	12,200	....
11. Church (Republican), Illinois—13th District, May 22, 1962, A3773	2,541	7,505	3,260
12. Cohelan (Democrat), California—7th District, June 23, 1962, A4773	10,659	5,338	1,003
13. Collier (Republican), Illinois—10th District, Mar. 29, 1961, A3846	2,700	5,310	990
14. Conte (Republican), Massachusetts—1st District, June 12, 1962, A4299	817	1,233	500
15. Corbett (Republican), Pennsylvania—29th District, Mar. 15, 1962, A1998	9,856	7,744	....
16. Derwinski (Republican), Illinois—4th District, May 14, 1962, p. 7643	7,920	21,780	3,300
17. Devine (Republican), Ohio—12th District, Mar. 29, 1962, A2482	1,352	4,454	511
18. Findley (Republican), Illinois—20th District, Mar. 28, 1962, p. 4929	3,395	5,607	....

19. Fisher (Democrat), Texas—21st District, Apr. 17, 1962, A2951	2,799	11,317	882
20. Frelinghuysen (Republican), New Jersey—5th District, May 24, 1961, A3701	4,240	3,120	640
21. Gathings (Democrat), Arkansas—1st District, May 8, 1961, A3163	480	960	60
22. Hall (Republican), Missouri—7th District, Apr. 16, 1962, A2905	2,148	8,688	1,164
23. Harvey (Republican), Indiana—10th District, May 3, 1962, A3286	456	1,387	72
24. Harvey (Republican), Michigan—8th District, June 18, 1962, A4583	1,407	2,823	1,471
25. Hiestand (Republican), California—21st District, May 10, 1962, A3476	5,400	10,800	1,800
26. Hosmer (Republican), California—18th District, June 26, 1961, A4766	4,240	3,280	480
27. Kastenmeier (Democrat), Wisconsin—2d District Apr. 19, 1962, A3083	1,777	1,412	....
28. Langen (Republican), Minnesota—9th District, May 2, 1962, p. 6957	2,178	6,435	1,287
29. Latta (Republican), Ohio—5th District, June 20, 1961, A4569	1,470	5,530	....
30. MacGregor (Republican), Minnesota—3d District, Jan. 10, 1962, A4	4,044	6,072	1,884
31. Martin (Republican), Nebraska—4th District, July 5, 1961, A5014	2,240	16,200	1,400
32. Mathias (Republican), Maryland—6th District, June 13, 1962, A4381	1,400	2,440	160
33. May (Republican), Washington—4th District, Feb. 26, 1962, A1382	7,204	10,903	1,362
34. Miller, Clem (Democrat), California—1st District, Oct. 10, 1962, A8099	8,330	7,140	1,530
35. Minshall (Republican), Ohio—23d District, Apr. 18, 1962, A3035	9,960	8,900	1,120
36. Monagan (Democrat), Connecticut—5th District, Apr. 17, 1962, A2948	957	504	334

37. Moorehead (Republican), Ohio—15th District, June 4, 1962, A4033	1,221	3,828	451
38. Ostertag (Republican), New York—39th District, Apr. 19, 1962, A3067	2,673	3,510	515
39. Pelly (Republican), Washington—1st District, Apr. 11, 1962, A2785	4,042	4,423	531
40. Pillion (Republican), New York—42d District, Apr. 18, 1962, A3001	2,774	3,389	....
41. Pirnie (Republican), New York—34th District, May 15, 1962, A3597	4,623	5,363	1,048
42. Proxmire (Democrat), Wisconsin—Senator, Sept. 18, 1961, p. 18, 755	1,202	798	....
43. Rogers (Democrat), Florida—6th District, May 17, 1961, A3482	26,612	21,774	....
44. Santangelo (Democrat), New York—18th District, May 4, 1961, A3130	3,700	1,300	....
45. Schneebeli (Republican), Pennsylvania—17th District, May 1, 1962, A3162	2,200	4,300	3,500
46. Shriver (Republican), Kansas—4th District, Aug. 1, 1961, A5898	884	1,870	145
47. Stratton (Democrat), New York—32d District, July 20, 1961, A5539	7,070	2,270	660
48. Toll (Democrat), Pennsylvania—6th District, June 22, 1962, A4731	2,250	672	78
49. Tollefson (Republican), Washington—6th District, Apr. 24, 1961, A2748	7,488	3,861	351
50. Van Zandt (Republican), Pennsylvania—20th District, Jan. 23, 1962, A412	863	1,731	....
51. Widnall (Republican), New Jersey—7th District, Aug. 23, 1961, A6630	7,500	4,500	....
52. Wilson (Republican), California—30th District Sept. 14, 1961, A7252	9,800	9,600	600
Total	241,383	334,399	39,502

Source: *Congressional Record,* July 10, 1962, p. 12177

Regarding the other important emphasis, the parliamentary question, nine opponents on fourteen occasions, and four supporters on four occasions, used it as an important debating point. The proponents argued that there were precedents for the attempt to originate the program in the Senate, and the opponents charged that it violated parliamentary procedures.

At this point it is well to discuss a tendency of the arguments of the stronger opponents to embrace ideas that fundamentally are in opposition to the principles of democratic theory. A colloquy between Senator Carl Curtis (R-Neb.) and Senator John O. Pastore (D-R.I.) supplies a concrete example. Senator Pastore asked Senator Curtis ". . . if the people of the United States want this program expanded after this beginning, what is so wrong about that? If the people of the United States . . . want this program, after they embark on it, to pay for more than hospitalization, what is wrong with that, if they want to pay for it?" To which Senator Curtis replied that the majority will is wrong, "because it will ruin the free practice of medicine in this country" (p. 11902).

Senator Allot also argued that the United States should not adopt the program, because "human beings are usually unwilling to pay for services given someone else as a right for long without insisting that right be extended also to them" (p. 12659). "Nor is public approval proof that a plan is good," he said, "this is particularly true in medical care." He supported this judgment by saying that "many people in England . . . seem to like their 'socialized medicine' " (p. 12660). Later in the very same argument he contradicted himself by saying that the people of Colorado, he was convinced, were almost unanimously opposed:

> . . . it is difficult for me to understand how this legislative body can even consider such a proposal as the one we have before us today, unless, we, too, are now willing to subscribe to the theory that this Government knows best what our people 'need', and, unless we are no longer interested in what they 'want' (p. 12668).

It would appear, therefore, that the majoritarian aspects of democratic theory are sound when they may be used to support one's position, but not otherwise. Incidentally, one of the reasons many supporters favor the use of the social security mechanism, both for the Old Age, Survivors, and Disability Insurance programs and for health benefits, is that it is "self-supporting," which means that it is not dependent upon annual appropriations by the Congress. This implies a certain measure of distrust of the legislative process by some supporters as well as by the more extreme opponents. So much for the ill-fated Anderson-Javits Amendment of 1962.

On July 6, 1965, Senator Long of Louisiana changed his position on health care and presented the Social Security amendments of 1965 (H.R. 6675) to the Senate. The bill proposed "to provide a hospital insurance program for the aged under the Social Security Act with a supplementary health benefits program and an expanded program of medical assistance, to increase benefits under the Old Age, Survivors, and Disability Insurance System, to improve the federal-state public assistance programs, and for other purposes." [7] Since there was no opposition to the increased social security benefits, the main point of controversy was Medicare, which would provide basic hospital protection to some nineteen million aged Americans and would establish a voluntary supplementary program to cover physicians' services and other health costs.

The Senate debate took place from July 6 to July 9, 1965. Fifty-one senators (thirty-eight supporters and thirteen opponents) participated in the debate which dominated the proceedings for the four-day period. Both supporters and opponents again presented their arguments in terms of certain basic American ideological themes, and again they employed similar concepts and symbols (private enterprise, American tradition, socialism). In comparing Table II (Analysis of the Senate Debate on the Anderson-Javits amendment) with Table III, however, it appears that, at the time of the H.R. 6675 debate, the use of rhetorical devices had diminished considerably, to be replaced by factual discussion and technical amendments. Though thirteen such devices continued to play an important part, the passage of Medicare apparently had been accepted by most senators as inevitable, reducing the elements of controversy, or at any rate making strenuous debating efforts hardly worthwhile.

Though the allusions to "American tradition" were not so emphatic as in the earlier debate, rhetorical appeal in this case was made primarily by supporters. When Senator Long introduced the bill, he said, "We are not . . . conforming with an international blueprint for social legislation. We are considering a bill which represents concern, consideration, and compromise in the best American tradition." [8]

TABLE II

ANALYSIS OF SENATE DEBATE ON
ANDERSON-JAVITS AMENDMENT

Number of Participants in the Debate: Supporters   26
   Opponents   19
   45

Major Debate Points	Supporters of Amendment		Opponents of Amendment	
	Number Using	Number of Times	Number Using	Number of Times
Conservatism	8	9	*	*
Insurance Mechanism	10	11	4	4
Private Enterprise	12**	28**	13	22
American Tradition	5	6	4	4
Socialism	11	17	9	13
British National Health Service	4	7	9	11
Other Foreign Systems	....	....	8	10
Parliamentary Procedure	4	4	9	14

*Used throughout the debates

**Number of Senators would be 13, and number of times would be 32 if discussion of the beneficial effects of the amendment upon private insurance companies were included.

TABLE III

ANALYSIS OF SENATE DEBATE ON
H.R. 6675 ("MEDICARE")

Number of Participants in the Debate:	Supporters	38
	Opponents	13
	Total	51

Major Debate Points	Supporters		Opponents	
	No. Using	No. of Times	No. Using	No. of Times
Conservatism	2	2	1	1
Insurance Mechanism	1	1	1	1
Private Enterprise	3	3	1	3
American Tradition	3	3	1	1
Socialism	2	2	3	5
British National Health Service	1	1	1	1
Other Foreign Systems	3	4	2	2

There were two points related to the "American tradition" argument which were used extensively by both sides in their attempts at "rhetorical reconciliation." First, supporters asserted that H.R. 6675 was purely an *American* plan. As illustrated by Senator Long's introduction in which he described the bill as the "democratic way of achieving social progress," the supporters presented the bill as a contrast to plans for "socialized medicine" in other countries.[9] That is, the Medicare provisions were presented as being uniquely American. Opponents, however, denied this because the bill provided coverage not only for those who needed it but also for those who were able to pay; in other words, all Americans aged sixty-five and above. The opposition argument, led by Senator Curtis, pivoted on this issue. Senator Curtis maintained that to provide medical care for the needy may well be within the American tradition. "It is not socialism for us to be charitable. . . . However, to pay the medical bills and hospital bills of individuals over sixty-five who are well able to provide the same for themselves is not charity. It is not needed. It is socialism." [10] Senator Curtis, therefore, presented the "American tradition" and "socialism" as being mutually exclusive. He further defined socialism as governmental aid to those who can pay their own way. Moreover, he asserted that to adopt such a program would represent a departure from "the private enterprise road that made us so great and strong." [11]

Subsequently he introduced an amendment to withhold Medicare from those who are able to pay. The ensuing controversy offers ample illustrations of distortions of language and "rhetorical reconciliation" on both sides of the question. Senator Frank Lausche (D-Ohio), for example, summarized the Curtis amendment as being un-American in that it imposed a greater burden on higher income groups and a lesser burden on lower income groups. In support of this stand, Senator Ribicoff declared that for all to pay equal amounts but then to receive benefits according to the amount of one's income is contrary to the principles of either private or social insurance. Nevertheless, several senators including Senator Russell Long who had earlier introduced a similar amendment in the committee, joined in support of the Curtis amendment. Their position was summarized by Senator Thruston Morton (R-Ky), who remarked that coverage for those able to pay "is certainly not the American way." [12]

The second argument used both by supporters and opponents related to the "dignity of the individual" and "independence." Proponents praised Medicare as a means of retaining the dignity of elderly persons by permitting economic independence. Senator Anderson in support of the bill said: "It is fitting that this nation should choose social insurance to assist its citizens in financing the high health costs that come with advancing years. For social insurance places its emphasis on that characteristic which distinguishes our free society from others—dignity of the individual. Social insurance rests on the principle that we Americans prize—that each should so far as possible pay his own way and be beholden to no one." [13] In contrast Senator Karl Mundt (R-S.D.) opposed the bill on the grounds that its passage "will be taking another step toward destroying the independence and self-reliance in America which is the last best hope of individual freedom for all mankind." [14]

With regard to "socialism" or "socialized medicine," the supporters tended to avoid the terms except to warn against them as scarewords, and to remind the Senate of the same cries that arose twenty-eight years earlier concerning the Social Security Act. Senator Moss, however, again viewed the measure as a means of forestalling "socialized medicine." As indicated by Table III, the opposition continued to stress charges of socialism but, because of the powerful support for the bill, all points received much less emphasis than in the Anderson-Javits debate. Three senators on five separate occasions warned against the danger. The height of emotional appeal is found in Senator Curtis's continual use of the term "socialism" as opposed to the private enterprise system. For example, he charged that "the enactment of this legislation is to turn our back upon private enterprise." The bill "is not only socialism—it is brazen socialism." [15]

The Curtis amendment was defeated fifty-one to forty-one. A later amendment to eliminate all Medicare provisions from H.R. 6675 was rejected sixty-four to twenty-six. A last attempt was made to introduce an alternate plan "better suited for our private enterprise system." When Senator Curtis was accused of using this as a delaying tactic, he replied that "it is a delaying action, in that it will delay the ultimate socialization of America." [16]

Two supporters on two occasions stressed the conservative nature of the bill, maintaining that it would not interfere with the practice of medicine or with the doctor-patient relationship, and would not bring about the socialization of America or destroy our private enterprise system. In praising the conservative mechanism of an insurance framework, Senator Thomas J.

McIntyre (D-N.H.) viewed the legislation as preserving "to the fullest the finest aspects of our national themes of free enterprise and freedom of choice." [17] Senator Moss maintained that the bill would enhance medical practice and the doctor-patient relationship by eliminating financial considerations. Three Senators proposed three plans for keeping the administration of the program on a local basis. Two of these plans advocated state administration by expanding the Kerr-Mills program. The third proposed that persons sixty-five and over receive payments from the government to pay for private insurance premiums.

The three remaining points on the table—insurance mechanism, the British National Health Service, and other foreign systems—were of little relevance in this debate. Only once did a supporting Senator allude to the insurance mechanism in praising the bill; only once did an opponent proclaim that social security measures are not truly based on a sound insurance principle. Four supporting senators on five different occasions referred to Britain's NHS or other foreign systems, but these allusions were mainly in presenting and debating technical amendments; though, as mentioned earlier, they implied that the bill was uniquely American. The three opponents who referred to the NHS or other foreign systems did so to illustrate the alleged dangers of Medicare. Two warned against the "approaching bankruptcy" of the welfare system in England and the "skyrocketing" taxes in other European countries. The third warned against a deterioration of our medical service.

As is apparent, the Anderson-Javits debate was the more significant of the two because it was more of a debate, and each side could anticipate the possibility, however remote, of victory and therefore made its greatest efforts.

There has been no attempt here to duplicate the excellent studies by Stephen K. Bailey and others of the internal intricacies of the congressional mechanism, or the thorough treatment by Donald R. Matthews of the United States Senate.[18]

This study serves merely to illustrate and to serve as a point of reference for certain of the arguments developed throughout this work. It deliberately ignores the findings of the experimental approach to the study of the legislative process not only because they are beyond the scope of this book, but also because there is a danger of misusing the materials of the behavioral sciences when moving from the laboratory to the "complex realities of the political scene." David B. Truman mentions the dangers involved in the reasoning by analogy that such a shift involves, and says that it is misleading or, at best, superficial.[19]

rhetorical reconciliation
and american leadership

The rhetorical reconciliation seems to apply equally to many phases of American society and is reflected in many ways. A look at American heroes and opinion regarding leadership within a democracy discloses a good illustration. An egalitarian system of beliefs should produce heroes who are accurate reflections of the people, who are able to fathom their wishes, and who speak and act as the people dictate. By the terms of the dominant American ideology, political heroes should be those who reflect the temper and wishes of the people.

In the United States, on the contrary, political heroes have tended to be manipulators of the public; men who are strong and effective as persons, not as spokesmen for what would now be called "public opinion." The ideology is a partial explanation for the well-known American deprecation of the "politician," and the rhetorical reconciliation is the device that transforms those who are most successful, on a sufficiently large scale, into "statesmen." The paradox is illustrated by an opinion survey that asked "would you like your son to go into politics?" and found that two-thirds of the respondents answered that they would not, and at the same time included a number of public offices at the top of their "value scales." [1]

Presidents who have used their power fully and effectively,

regardless of their platforms or parties, have been rewarded with favorable public sentiment as well as by the "verdict of history." In spite of anti-governmental attitudes, when crises have threatened, the government has received the authority necessary to deal with the emergency. The reluctance to yield power until it cannot be avoided without catastrophe probably results in greater governmental activity than if the power were not so jealously guarded. A more energetic government during relatively normal periods might have been able to prevent some of the more severe crises that have necessitated rather extensive grants of power to the government.

During the Great Depression, the people cried out for leadership. They had no carefully formulated plans for action; they had merely a desire for a strong leader who could effectively combat the economic disasters. Their choice, Franklin D. Roosevelt, become simultaneously one of a small group of presidents who exercised power most forcefully, and probably the greatest American cultural hero of the twentieth century.

Even writers not overly friendly to Roosevelt and the New Deal admit that the people sought nothing so much as leadership. According to the historian Edgar E. Robinson, the dominant feeling during the 1934 congressional elections was gratitude to the President for his leadership.[2] He says, correctly, that millions of Americans considered Roosevelt their savior, but says also that the President's leadership was "injurious to the slow working of democracy as Americans know it, and have thought of it in terms of the leadership of Jefferson or Lincoln or Wilson." [3] He does not define the leadership of Jefferson or Lincoln or Wilson, but criticizes FDR for reliance upon unofficial advisers, with subsequent "arbitrary and personal" decisions. Although Robinson evidently defines leadership as good when based upon the advice of "official advisers" and bad if based upon the counsel of "unofficial advisers," he agrees that leadership was the prime quality the people demanded, and was the major reason for their gratitude to Roosevelt. As late as 1940, Harold L. Ickes writes that the President could have lost "a million votes a week" if the people had concluded that his leadership had not been firm, understanding, and forward looking.[4]

The charisma of the President contributed greatly to the changes in the society produced by the depression. One of the most significant changes was in the realm of political behavior. Since the Civil War, for example, the Negro vote had been heavily Republican. Roy Wilkins of the National Association for the Advancement of Colored People has been quoted as saying that in his childhood, "kids threw rocks at Negroes on our street who dared to vote Democratic." [5] Likewise, Representative William Dawson from Chicago, who had been raised in Georgia and taught to hate the word "Democrat," describes his switch from the Republican party during the depression. Speaking not of the New Deal but of Roosevelt, Dawson said "Negroes would have died like flies if he hadn't kept his hand on the money until it got to them." Dawson went on to become a Democratic political boss, one of many such men who have come to exercise considerable power, both as local bosses and as those capable of delivering large numbers of the Negro votes which are now so influential in national politics.[6]

Although the effect was more dramatic upon the minority groups, the country as a whole was actively seeking to be led. Roosevelt was the only strong leader known to the public as seeking democratic reform. Ickes says that this was the reason for his success, that the people saw the President as the only one in a position to give them national leadership.[7]

Regardless of the American distrust of politicians and the executive, the United States has traditionally honored those executives capable of firm and decisive action. The Presidents who have adhered to the conception of the separation of powers, and have confined their roles to the acceptance or rejection of legislation are, in the words of D. W. Brogan, those "whom American tradition has least delighted to honour." [8] As the office has grown, it has taken on even more symbolism and has extended its charismatic character.

The governmental system was established deliberately to reduce the energy of the government, and to prevent the exercise, not only of arbitrary power, but simply of power; yet those executives who have been most successful in circumventing the restrictions upon the exercise of power have become cultural heroes. Since the system in operation is one of balance and a maintenance of the *status quo*, the most energetic executives have been those who have pressed for social change. It is paradoxical that, in a nation characteristically exhibiting little receptivity toward new social ideas and other expressions of nonconformity, those most honored tend to be the agents of social change.

The American ideology includes an aversion to the exercise of power; but, in practice, the people tend to accept the person capable of an exercise of power beyond the limits established by the ideology; the public actually seems to have a high regard for the successful exercise of power, even though it theoretically abhors it. Obviously, the pragmatic temper of the people and their ideology often are in conflict. The ideology often delays or perhaps restrains action, but rarely prevents it. The British observers Hugh-Jones and Radice noted in the 1930's that the Democratic party has traditionally been the representative of the Jeffersonian position; the Republican, that of Hamilton; yet it has been largely through Democratic Presidents from "Jefferson himself, through Jackson, Cleveland, and Wilson, down to F. D. Roosevelt, that the Federal power has been steadily extended." [9]

Though this ignores Lincoln and Theodore Roosevelt, the point is a good one: ideology does not govern practice. The ideology, however, is tenacious, hence the necessity of a reconciliation between contradictory practices and beliefs. The rhetorical solution has enabled Americans to accomplish this; it has permitted the ideology to exist simultaneously with that which is, in practice, a worship of success. That the admiration is for success, as opposed to social change, per se, is evidenced by the status of military leaders. These men are admired for their success, and for their apparently firm decisive actions even though they take their actions within the framework of the most authoritarian segment of adult America (excepting that within correctional institutions).

The social theorist Hans L. Zetterberg concludes that the dilemma of democracies is their tendency to elect to office, in times of crisis, those who work to retain an unsatisfactory *status quo*.[10] During "ordinary" times it seems true that this tendency may exist. A glance at periods of crisis in American history, however, indicates that Zetterberg's conception of the "democratic dilemma" has not characterized the United States. Throughout American history, periods of extreme crisis have brought forth powerful leaders whose strategies involved action rather than attempts specifically to restore former conditions. The Revolution, the Civil War, the Great Depression (leading into World War II), and perhaps the first World War were the most severe crises in the history of this country; during each, the public chose leaders of the highest stature whose interests did not concern mainly the preservation of the *status quo*.

During the Great Depression, for example, the people elected Franklin D. Roosevelt, who established policies and recommended action programs with little regard for tradition. As late as 1948, a poll by Elmo Roper found that 43% listed FDR when asked "out of all the men in America who have been prominent in public affairs during the past 50 years, which one or two have you admired the most?" [11] This frank admiration for the strong leader, for the man who is successful in his exercise of power, contradicts an ideology of egalitarianism, but is consistent with the pragmatic temper of the people.

The fundamental American pragmatism has encouraged the separation of ideology from reality by emphasizing action as opposed to thought. With the supremacy of action, the ideology has been able to survive with little revision so that it retains many features that are anachronistic. This has led to its increasing sterility as it becomes less relevant to practice. The espoused principles of modern "conservatism" present an excellent example.

Jasper B. Shannon of the University of Nebraska has analyzed conservative thought and says that its political strategy is to equate the exercise of governmental power with the old tyrannical power of a monarch. Since modern conservatism does not approve of the concentration of power in public governments, popular consent does not justify the exercise of governmental power. Conservatives, in the name of free enterprise, may approve of the exercise, through concentrated power in the economy, of economic sovereignty over the lives of millions of people, but shift the argument from economics to individual liberty when the government exercises power.[12]

If this is an accurate description of conservative thought as it is expressed in America, conservative thought is largely irrelevant. These principles guide very few people in this country. Both liberals and conservatives have encouraged government action in the economy on pragmatic grounds since the beginnings of industrialism. The reaction to a government program tends to be based not upon abstract considerations regarding the exercise of power, but upon the predicted effect upon the various segments of the society. Shannon's general observation that the symbols of "free enterprise" and "individual liberty" are used inconsistently to justify and condemn, according to the issue involved, is, of course, unquestionable.

There is another side to the traditional American acceptance of strong leaders, contrary to ideological bias. In the political sphere, it is manifested by the popular acclaim given to strong Presidents; in the intellectual sphere, the same tendency may be seen in the typical American reliance upon "experts." D. W. Brogan notes a "democratic inertia" that is especially prominent in the United States, with the typical American considering himself extraordinarily self-reliant, yet eager to follow leaders and to turn his problems over to "experts" and "organizations." [13] A reliance upon an expert is convenient as a method for avoiding active thought and for evading responsibility.

The marked antipathy toward the intellectual or the "egghead" in American culture does not prevent the public from an acceptance of the symbol of "Science" or a reliance upon anything that purports to be scientific. This has been influenced by the prevailing activist, or pragmatic, view. American culture traditionally has tended to respect action and ignore theory, resulting in a narrowing of intellectual experience for the typical citizen. Without a breadth of intellectual interest, the American tends to give credence to those who allege competence in subjects outside his range of activity, especially if the subjects are characterized by formidable technical terms and other manifestations of the mysterious. Except for scientists, the "experts" rarely are theoreticians or "eggheads" but are men of action whose appeal to the pragmatic American is immediate.

Practitioners of the modern scientific disciplines have accomplished many feats that seem almost miraculous. The jargon of the sciences, therefore, when applied or misapplied to any issue, tends to invest the position advanced with an aura of infallibility, so that Americans tend to accept statements called "scientific" with little question. In social matters, the use of scientific techniques to infer "laws" or to assume a predictive certainty ignores the role of human intelligence. So great has been the tendency to accept all applications of Science that belief in a new determinism, although unacknowledged as such, renders incredible the simultaneously held belief in the primacy of the individual.[14]

The passive acceptance of "Science" and the scientific terminology does not entirely explain the American predilection for subordinating thought processes to those of experts—often self-appointed experts without the faintest hint of a qualification. A case in point is the extraordinary popularity of the "advice to the love-lorn" columns in the daily newspapers.

Frequently, even these are clothed with pseudo-scientific terminology. Similar in its acceptance, but without the scientific implications, is the status accorded the authority upon etiquette. Although the American ostensibly rejects authoritarianism, he tends to subjects himself without question to dictates from on high concerning dress, conduct, health, and even the fathoming of his personality and capabilities.

The lack of concern with intellectual matters and the acceptance of symbols, the results of polls, and other manufactured opinions in lieu of critical thought, are capable of combining with admiration for strong leaders to produce a climate in which the public may be receptive to direction. The two major demagogues of the 1930's, Father Coughlin and Huey Long (not to mention the demagogic traditions of the South, or the followings of those who have devoted themselves in the last few decades to the suppression of "deviant" political opinion) proved that wide segments of the society will at times support political figures whose tactics, and even whose programs, are explicitly opposed to democratic theory and the dominant ideology. Significantly, however, without regard to the content of his programs, the American demagogue has typically appealed to the people in the language of democracy.

Although the United States has never, for any length of time, wholeheartedly accepted the demagogue, it has had its dangerous periods, and the danger is increased by the tendency to resort to the "rhetorical reconciliation." The one true safeguard, a sound body of principles that guide action, does not exist if the public tends to accept a sterile ideology and is accustomed to the adoption of practices contrary to that ideology without recognizing the conflict.

"Rhetorical reconciliations" can lead to the acceptance of practices that violate the ideological tenets of political and civil liberties, just as easily as they can lead to the acceptance of programs violating the tenets of laissez-faire economics. With all due regard for the tendency for Americans to accept strong leaders when there is a need for action, there is perhaps a greater danger that the society itself, through a tendency to accept uncritically the forces that manipulate it, can impose a dictatorship, perhaps an apolitical dictatorship, as severe as that under a frankly authoritarian political order.

Throughout the entire range of contemporary American public experience, it is possible to observe the influence of the rhetorical reconciliation. From education to entertainment, from city life to civil rights, from the military to the marketplace, its effects are evident. The American can retain his ideology of democracy and individualism, yet can worship the strong and powerful leader; he can retain the ideology of resourcefulness and self-reliance, yet abdicate many of his opinion-forming thought processes to "experts" and public-opinion polls, both of which are indispensable in modern society but are misused when they supply pre-conceived positions upon a range of subjects; he can retain an ideology of equality, yet seek actively to rise above his fellow men in a society characterized by an inequality that is real, even though it may be less than in many other societies, and is mollified by welfare programs, social insurance, and other government activities as well as by a strong and vigorous economy. The major reconciliation of opposites that permits the American to live at peace with practices directly contrary to his ideology, is largely rhetorical.

notes

I THE AMERICAN IDEOLOGY

1. David Potter, *People of Plenty: Economic Abundance and the American Character* (Chicago: University of Chicago Press, 1954), p. 123.

2. Ibid., pp. 137–138.

3. Clinch Calkins, *Some Folks Won't Work* (New York: Harcourt Brace, and World, 1930) pp. 19–21.

4. E. M. Hugh-Jones and E. A. Radice, *An American Experiment* (London: Oxford University Press, 1936), p. 174. Hugh-Jones, an Oxford economist, spent the years 1933 and 1934 travelling in the United States as a Rockefeller Fellow. Radice, also of Oxford, was in this country from 1933 to 1935 under the auspices of the Commonwealth Fund.

5. Karl Mannheim, *Diagnosis of Our Time* (New York: Oxford University Press, 1944), Preface to the American Edition, p. vii.

6. Potter, pp. 8–11.

7. Ibid., p. 65

8. Henry Steele Commager, *The American Mind: An Interpretation of American Thought and Character Since the 1880's* (New Haven: Yale University Press, 1950), p. 1.

9. Ibid., p. 409.

10. Reuel Denney, "How Americans See Themselves," in *Studies in American Culture,* Joseph Kwiat and Mary Turpie, eds. (Minneapolis: University of Minnesota Press, 1960), pp. 19–20.

11. Commager, pp. 314–315.

12. Ibid., p. 406.

13. Harvey Wish, *Society and Thought in Modern America* (New York: Longmans, Green, & Co., 1953) , p. 493.

14. William E. Leuchtenburg, *Franklin D. Roosevelt and The New Deal, 1932–1940* (New York: Harper & Row, Publishers, 1963) , p. 165.

15. Robert S. and Helen Merrell Lynd, *Middletown: A Study in American Culture* (New York: Harcourt, Brace, and World, 1956) , p. 88 (originally published in 1929) .

16. Max Lerner, *America as a Civilization* (New York: Simon & Schuster, 1957) , p. 339.

17. Sherwood Anderson, *Puzzled America* (New York: Charles Scribner's Sons, 1935) , p. 46.

18. Potter, p. 93.

19. Ida C. Merriam, "Trends in Public Welfare and Their Implications," *American Economic Review*, XLVII (May 1957) , pp. 480–481.

20. Committee on Economic Security, *Social Security in America, The Background of the Social Security Act as Summarized from Staff Reports to the Committee on Economic Security* (Washington: U. S. Government Printing Office, 1937) , Chapter VII.

21. Robert and Helen Lynd, *Middletown*, p. 59.

22. Irving Bernstein, *The Lean Years, A History of the American Worker, 1920–1933* (Boston: Houghton Mifflin Co., 1960) , pp. 59–63; for examples of the personal consequences of unemployment see Helen Hall, *Case Studies of Unemployment* (Philadelphia: University of Pennsylvania Press, 1931) .

23. Joanna C. Colcord, "The Challenge of the Continuing Depression," *Annals*, American Academy of Political and Social Science, CLXXVI (November 1934) , p. 16.

24. Hugh-Jones and Radice, p. 44.

25. Thurmon Arnold, *The Symbols of Government* (New Haven: Yale University Press, 1935) , p. 121.

26. Leuchtenburg, p. 132.

27. Arnold, p. 121.

28. Robert and Helen Lynd, *Middletown in Transition* (New York: Harcourt, Brace, and World, 1937) , p. 72. This is the second pioneer community study of Muncie, Indiana that the Lynds conducted.

29. Frederick Lewis Allen, "Economic Security: A Look Back and a Look Ahead," *Economic Security for Americans* (New York: The American Assembly, 1954) , p. 14.

30. *Middletown in Transition,* p. 490.

31. Ibid., p. 502

32. Commager, p. 354.

33. William Whyte, *The Organization Man* (New York: Simon & Schuster, 1956), p. 355.

34. Art Gallaher, Jr., *Plainville Fifteen Years Later* (New York: Columbia University Press, 1961), Introduction.

35. James West (Carl Withers, pseud.), *Plainville, U.S.A.* (New York: Columbia University Press, 1945), p. 216.

36. Ibid., p. 30.

37. Gallaher, p. 35.

38. Ibid., p. 90.

39. Ibid., pp. 128–129.

40. Ibid., pp. 255–256.

41. Lerner, p. 355.

42. American Assembly, *Economic Security for Americans* (New York, 1954), p. 7.

43. John Kenneth Galbraith, *The Affluent Society* (Cambridge, Massachusetts: The Riverside Press, 1958), p. 99.

II THE AMERICAN PROCESS OF RHETORICAL RECONCILIATION

1. Vilfredo Pareto, *The Mind and Society: A Treatise on General Sociology*, Arthur Livingston, ed. (New York: Harcourt, Brace, and World, 1963), pp. 508–511 (Italian edition 1923; first U.S. edition 1935).

2. Ibid., p. 899.

3. Ibid., p. 1202.

4. Karl Mannheim, *Essays on the Sociology of Culture*, Ernest Manheim, ed. (New York: Oxford University Press, 1956), p. 178 (also see footnote).

5. William W. Biddle, *Propaganda and Education* (New York: Columbia University Press, 1932), pp. 1–3.

6. Commager, p. 420.

7. Potter, pp. 187–188.

8. Mannheim, *Essays,* p. 178.

9. Aldous Huxley, *Brave New World Revisited* (New York: Harper & Row, 1958), p. 33.

10. Ibid., p. 103.

11. Reprinted in *Identity and Anxiety: Survival of the Person in Mass Society,* Stein et al, eds. (Glencoe, Illinois: The Free Press of Glencoe, 1960), pp. 308–319.

12. Ibid.

13. C. K. Ogden and I. A. Richards, *The Meaning of Meaning* (New York: Harcourt, Brace, and World, 1963), p. 25.

14. Louis Hartz, *The Liberal Tradition in America* (New York: Harcourt, Brace, and World, 1955), p. 205.

15. Jerome Frank, "A Lawyer Looks at Language," in S. I. Hayakawa, *Language in Action* (New York: Harcourt, Brace, and World, 1940), p. 326.

16. Stephen K. Bailey, *Congress Makes A Law: The Story Behind the Unemployment Act of 1946* (New York: Columbia University Press, 1950), p. 46.

17. J. Douglas Brown, "The Role of Social Insurance in the United States," *Industrial and Labor Relations Review,* XIV (October 1960), pp. 107–112.

18. Herman and Anne Somers, "Social Security in the United States of America: Recent Development and Emerging Concepts," *Bulletin of the International Social Security Association,* X (March–April 1957), p. 88.

19. George W. Hartmann, "The Contradiction Between the Feeling-Tone of Political Party Names and Public Response to Their Platforms," *Journal of Social Psychology,* VII (August 1936), p. 339.

20. See chapter IX, "The Language of Learning and of Pedantry," in Jacques Barzun's, *The House of Intellect* (New York: Harper Torchbooks, 1959), for an incisive discussion of the state of the language.

21. Stuart Chase, *The Tyranny of Words* (New York: Harcourt, Brace, and World, 1938), pp. 353–354.

22. Quoted by Stuart Chase in *Guides to Straight Thinking* (New York: Harper & Row, 1956), p. 193.

23. Commager, p. 341.

24. Thurman Arnold, *The Folklore of Capitalism* (New Haven: Yale University Press, 1937), pp. 380–381.

25. John Kenneth Galbraith, "The Age of the Wordfact," *The Atlantic Monthly,* CCVI (September, 1960), pp. 87–90.

26. Friedrich A. Hayek, *The Road to Serfdom* (Chicago: University of Chicago Press, 1957), p. 37.

27. Ibid., pp. 119–120.

28. Daniel Bell, *The End of Ideology* (Glencoe, Illinois: The Free Press of Glencoe, 1957), p. 73.

29. Quoted in A. T. Mason, ed., *Free Government in the Making* (New York: Oxford University Press, 1956), pp. 804–806.

30. John P. Roche, *The Quest for the Dream: The Development*

of Civil Rights and Human Relations in Modern America (New York: Macmillan Co., 1963), p. 135.

31. Graham Hutton, "Utopia is No Bargain," *Journal of American Insurance,* XXXVIII (September 1962), p. 5.

32. "America—Beware . . . ," p. 2 (AMA information pamphlet).

33. Ibid., p. 3.

34. Hans Zetterberg, *Social Theory and Social Practice* (New York: The Bedminster Press, 1962), p. 16, footnote.

35. Quoted by Stephen K. Bailey, "New Research Frontiers of Interest to Legislators and Administrators," in *Research Frontiers in Politics and Government: Brookings Lectures, 1955* (Washington: The Brookings Institution, 1955), p. 15.

III   THE SOCIAL SECURITY ACT AND THE "INSURANCE COMPANY MODEL"

1. Ralph E. and Muriel W. Pumphrey, eds., *The Heritage of American Social Work* (New York: Columbia University Press, 1961), p. 319.

2. Clarke A. Chambers, *Seedtime of Reform* (Minneapolis: University of Minnesota Press, 1963), pp. 3–11.

3. I. M. Rubinow, *Social Insurance* (New York: Henry Holt & Co., 1913), p. 6.

4. Chambers, p. 89.

5. See Odin W. Anderson, "Compulsory Medical Care Insurance, 1910–1950," *Annals,* American Academy of Political and Social Science, CCLXXIII (January 1951), pp. 106–113.

6. Ibid.

7. I. M. Rubinow, *Standards of Health Insurance* (New York: Henry Holt & Co., 1916).

8. Anderson, pp. 106–113.

9. Chambers, pp. 171–172.

10. Paul H. Douglas, *Wages and the Family* (Chicago: University of Chicago Press, 1925).

11. Chambers, p. 158.

12. John D. Hicks, *Republican Ascendancy* (New York: Harper & Row, 1960), p. 73.

13. Irving Bernstein, *The Lean Years, A History of the American Worker, 1920–1933* (Boston: Houghton Mifflin Co., 1960), p. 237.

14. Paul Douglas, *Social Security in the United States* (New York: McGraw-Hill Book Co., 1939), p. 5.

15. Ibid.; the eight states were Colorado, Kentucky, Maryland, Montana, Minnesota, Nevada, Utah, and Wisconsin. California and

Wyoming, in 1929, were the first to adopt mandatory acts. New York and Massachusetts followed in 1930, Colorado (replacing the old act) ; Delaware, Idaho, New Jersey, and New Hampshire followed in 1931; and Arizona, Indiana, Maine, Michigan, Nebraska, North Dakota, Ohio, Oregon, Pennsylvania, and Washington joined the list in 1933. By the middle of 1934, twenty-eight states plus Alaska and Hawaii had passed old age pension acts, all but five of them mandatory Ibid., pp. 5–7) .

16. Chambers, p. 33.

17. Ibid., p. 40.

18. Ibid., pp. 93–180.

19. Bernstein, p. 475.

20. Abraham Epstein, *Insecurity: A Challenge to America* (New York: Harrison Smith & Robert Haas, Inc., 1936), revised edition, pp. 22–23.

21. Ibid., p. 35.

22. Ibid., p. 43.

23. Rubinow, *The Quest for Security* (New York: Holt, Rinehart & Winston, Inc., 1934), pp. 520–521.

24. Arthur M. Schlesinger, Jr., *The Age of Roosevelt: The Coming of the New Deal* (Boston: Houghton Mifflin Co., 1959), p. 298.

25. Bernstein, p. 475.

26. Pumphrey, p. 439 (footnote).

27. See Douglas, *Social Security in the United States,* chapter IV, for an excellent legislative history of the Social Security Act.

28. See *Social Security Programs Throughout the World,* U. S. Department of Health, Education, and Welfare: Social Security Administration, 1961, *passim.*

29. Committee on Economic Security, *Social Security in America, The Background of the Social Security Act as Summarized from Staff Reports to the Committee on Economic Security* (Washington: U. S. Government Printing Office, 1937), pp. 212–213.

30. Rubinow, *Quest,* pp. 287–301.

31. Epstein, pp. 761–765.

32. Schlesinger, p. 310.

33. Committee on Economic Security, p. 89–90.

34. The information on party platforms is from Kirk Porter and Donald Johnson, *National Party Platforms, 1840–1956* (Urbana, Illinois: University of Illinois Press, 1956) .

35. *New York Times,* May 8, 1936.

36. Washington *Post,* June 10, 1936.

37. *New York Times,* November 1, 1936.

38. Franklin D. Roosevelt, *Selected Speeches, Messages, Press Conferences, and Letters,* Basil Rauch, ed. (New York: Holt, Rinehart & Winston, Inc., 1957) , pp. 161–165.

39. Robert and Helen Lynd, *Middletown in Transition,* p. 361.

40. Washington *Herald,* May 28, 1936.

41. New York *Herald Tribune,* September 29, 1936.

42. Ibid., November 2, 1936.

43. *New York Times,* August 30, 1936.

44. Ibid., December 30, 1939.

45. *Collier's,* November 28, 1936, p. 66.

46. *New York Times,* May 8, 1936.

47. See, e.g., V. O. Key, Jr., *Politics, Parties and Pressure Groups* (New York: Thomas Y. Crowell & Co., 1953) , 3rd edition, p. 205.

48. See *Congressional Record,* 74th Congress, 1st session, pp. 9648–9650 and 6069–6070.

49. V. O. Key, Jr., *Public Opinion and American Democracy* (New York: Alfred A. Knopf, Inc., 1961) , p. 31.

50. For a summary of major polls throughout the world on many subjects, see *Public Opinion, 1935–1946,* Hadley Cantril, ed. (Princeton: Princeton University Press, 1951) .

51. Douglas, p. 1.

52. Cantril, p. 541.

53. Ibid.

54. Ibid., p. 542.

55. Elmo Roper, *You and Your Leaders: Their Actions and Your Reactions, 1936–1956* (New York: William Morrow & Co., 1957) , p. 61.

56. Ibid., p. 193.

57. C. A. Kulp, "American Provisions for Old-Age Security," *Annals,* American Academy of Political and Social Science, CCII (March 1939) , p. 69.

58. See, for example, the testimony of Arthur Altmeyer (who had been the first Commissioner for Social Security) before a subcommittee of the House Ways and Means Committee, *Analysis of the Social Security System,* 83rd Congress, first session, 1953, Part 6, pp. 879–1015, *passim.*

59. Schlesinger, p. 310.

60. Leuchtenburg, *Franklin D. Roosevelt . . . ,* p. 132.

61. Edwin Witte, *The Development of the Social Security Act* (Madison: University of Wisconsin Press, 1962) , p. 173; Witte was the executive director of the Committee on Economic Security and,

in 1936, produced the confidential memorandum (now on file in the Social Security Administration Library, Baltimore) upon which his book is based.

62. Ibid., p. viii.

63. Ibid., p. 176.

64. Ibid., p. 177.

65. Ibid., pp. 177–180.

66. Ibid., pp. 180–181.

67. Ibid., pp. 181–189.

68. *JAMA,* Dec. 3, 1932, p. 1950.

69. Oliver Garceau, "Organized Medicine Enforces its 'Party Line,' " *Public Opinion Quarterly,* IV (September 1940), p. 408; the quotation from Van Etten appeared originally in an editorial in *JAMA,* June 22, 1940, p. 2472.

70. Quoted in U. S. Chamber of Commerce, *American Economic Security,* Special Issue, Proceedings of the third National Conference on Social Security of March 31, 1949, April–May 1949, p. 72.

71. Resolution by Eugene E. Hoffman at the Clinical Session, December, 1951; see *Proceedings,* pp. 70 and 80–81.

72. See *American Medical Association News,* October 28, 1963, p. 5.

73. Garceau, p. 409.

74. See "The American Medical Association: Power, Purpose and Politics in Organized Medicine," *Yale Law Journal,* LXIII (May 1954), p. 1015, footnote 659 (hereafter referred to as *Yale Law Journal*).

75. "Doctors Hit AMA Ban of Ad for Aged Care," Washington *Star,* May 17, 1962.

76. David Rutstein, "The Medical Care Pork Barrel," *The Atlantic Monthly,* CCVII (March 1961), pp. 61–64; letter from T. A. Dippy, June 1961, p. 32.

IV MEDICARE

1. Morris Fishbein, *A History of the American Medical Association* (Philadelphia: W. B. Sounders Co., 1947), pp. 318–321.

2. Anderson, *loc. cit.*

3. Fishbein, *loc. cit.*

4. For excellent summaries of proposed federal health-insurance legislation, see Agnes W. Brewster, *Health Insurance and Related Proposals for Financing Personal Health Services* (Washington: U.S. Department of Health, Education, and Welfare: Social Security

Administration, 1958), and *The Yale Law Journal*, esp. pp. 1007–1018; the description of the propaganda campaign through 1953 relies primarily upon the *Yale Law Journal*.

5. *Yale Law Journal*, p. 1008.

6. Ibid., p. 1009; esp. footnote 602.

7. Ibid.

8. Ibid.

9. Ibid., pp. 1011–1014.

10. Ibid., p. 1016.

11. Ibid., p. 1017; see footnote 676.

12. *New York Times*, January 18, 1962. p. 1.

13. Based on interviews with health insurance executives conducted by the author during 1961–1962.

14. "Companies Press Health Policies," *New York Times*, January 6, 1964, p. 12.

15. "Aged Care Action is Expected Today," *New York Times*, Sept. 30, 1964, p. 17.

16. "Mills Gives Way on Aged Care Bill," *New York Times*, November 12, 1964, p. 1.

17. "Movement on Medicare?" (Editorial) *New York Times*, November 13, 1964, p. 34.

18. "New Health Plan Offered by A.M.A.," *New York Times*, January 10, 1966, p. 1.

19. The two Democrats voting against the measure were Representatives Herlong and John C. Watts (Kentucky).

V THE BATTLE

1. *JAMA*, July 21, 1962, p. 265.

2. *PR Reporter*, May 28, 1962, pp. 1–2; this publication describes itself as "a working newsletter for public relations professionals."

3. Ibid.

4. Ibid.

5. See "We Support Health Benefits for the Aged through Social Security," *National Association of Social Workers* (New York, 1961) for a list of organizations and prominent persons supporting the bill.

6. U.S. Congress, *Health Services for the Aged Under the Social Security Insurance System*, Hearings before the Ways and Means Committee (Washington, U.S. Government Printing Office, 1961), pp. 701–702 (cited hereafter as "Hearings").

7. The Blue Shield plans, on the other hand, are generally

creatures of state medical societies; the national Blue Shield organization is closely allied with the American Medical Association and separate from the Blue Cross Association.

8. Richard Hofstadter, *The Paranoid Style in American Politics, and Other Essays* (New York: Alfred A. Knopf, Inc., 1965).

9. In this regard it should be noted that the first months after passage of the Medicare Bill in 1965, many individuals and a number of local groups let it be known that they would not treat patients under Medicare. Attempts to persuade the American Medical Association to make such refusals binding on the membership were unsuccessful, but the idea was seriously considered.

10. Wayne G. Menke, "The Doctor: Change and Conflict in American Medical Practice," unpublished Ph.D. thesis, University of Minnesota, 1961, p. 294.

11. Center for the Study of Democratic Institutions, *Medicine: An Interview by Donald McDonald with Herbert Ratner, M.D.,* Santa Barbara, California, 1962, pp. 3–4.

12. "Does the U.S. Really Have the World's Finest Medical Care?" *Consumer Reports,* March 1965, pp. 146–150; for other material see the critical study by Roul Tunley, *The American Health Scandal* (New York: Harper & Row, 1966); for a contrary view, see the attack upon the critics by Representative Thomas B. Curtis, "The United States has the Best Medical and Health Services in the World," Congressional Record, March 17, 1966, pp. 5922–5929.

13. "Hearings," p. 163.

14. See statement of Howard Phillips, member, board of directors, Young Americans for Freedom, before the House Ways & Means Committee; "Hearings," p. 751.

15. Copyright 1962 by *The Independent American,* Kent Courtney, Publisher, Phoebe Courtney, Editor.

16. Michigan Health Council, East Lansing, Michigan, Copyright, 1961.

17. "British Record Supplement to British Record No. 1," Jan. 15, 1962.

18. Weldon Wallace, "Fight Socialism, Physicians Told," Baltimore *Sun,* Sept. 15, 1961, p. 28.

19. Joan Graham, "Dr. Varley's View of English Doctors, Clergymen is Hit," Baltimore *Sun,* September 19, 1961, p. 38.

20. *British Medical Journal,* July 14, 1962, p. 105.

21. Trenton *Evening Times,* May 8, 1962.

22. Ibid.

23. "Congressman Thompson's Report," Trenton *Trentonian,* May 9, 1962.

24. Trenton *Trentonian,* May 10, 1962.

25. New Brunswick *Sunday Home News,* May 13, 1962.

26. For an excellent brief summary of the structure and activities of the AMA, including what is known of AMPAC, see Austin C. Wehrwein, "A.M.A. is Continuing Fight Against Medical Care Bill," *New York Times,* October 18, 1964, p. 76.

27. For an example of this advertisement, see the *New York Times,* June 9, 1965, p. 36.

28. Quoted in "Doctors Pressed to Defy Medicare," *New York Times,* June 19, 1965, p. 30.

29. "Dr. Fishbein Says Conditions Change, He Is for Medicare," *New York Times,* October 30, 1965.

VI RHETORICAL RECONCILIATION IN THE U.S. SENATE

1. See S. 3565, Eighty-Seventh Congress, pp. 45–59.

2. See *Congressional Record,* Eighty-Seventh Congress, second session, July 17, 1962, daily edition, pp. 12924–12925; the numbers in parentheses in this section refer to page numbers in the *Record.*

3. Washington *Post,* November 15, 1963, p. A4.

4. Thirty-five senators reported to the author that they received more mail about Medicare than on "other questions of significant interest"; fifteen reported that the mail was "about the same" (relatively heavy) and two reported having received less. Studies of congressional mail support the contention that the political approach of the public is pragmatic and that citizens tend to be concerned with specific issues affecting them at the expense of their devotion to general principles. See Bailey, *Congress at Work* (New York: Holt, Rinehart & Winston, Inc., 1952) , pp. 99–102, for an analysis of Senator Lehman's mail during a six-month period in 1951, including a tabulation for one day; and see Donald R. Matthews, *U.S. Senators and their World* (Chapel Hill: University of North Carolina Press, 1960) for a good general discussion of the subject. Also valuable for examples of congressional mail is Estes Kefauver and J. Levin, *A Twentieth-Century Congress* (New York: Essential Books, 1947) , Chapter 13.

5. See, for example, Senator Anderson's statement on p. 12723, "Yes Mr. President, fortunately the responsible, conservative way to finance the program is also the popular way. . . ."

6. Matthews, p. 223, footnote; see also Harry Alpert, et al, "Con-

gressional Use of Polls: A Symposium," *Public Opinion Quarterly,* XVIII (Summer, 1954) , pp. 121–142.

7. *Congressional Record,* Eighty-Ninth Congress, first session, July 6, 1965, p. 15037.

8. Ibid.

9. Ibid.

10. Ibid., July 8, 1965, p. 15298.

11. Ibid., p. 15301.

12. Ibid., p. 15307.

13. Ibid., July 6, 1965, pp. 15065–15066.

14. Ibid., July 9, 1965, p. 15552.

15. Ibid., July 8, 1965, p. 15299.

16. Ibid., July 9, 1965, pp. 15549–15550.

17. Ibid., p. 15577.

18. See Bailey's *Congress Makes a Law,* and his *Congress at Work;* Matthews; David B. Truman's *The Governmental Process* (New York: Alfred A. Knopf, 1951) ; and his *The Congressional Party: A Case Study* (New York: John B. Wiley & Sons, 1959) .

19. David B. Truman, "The Impact on Political Science of the Revolution in the Behavioral Sciences," in *Research Frontiers in Politics.*

VII   Rhetorical Reconciliation and American Leadership

1. Stuart Chase, *American Credos* (New York: Harper & Row, Inc., 1962) , p. 117.

2. Edgar E. Robinson, *The Roosevelt Leadership, 1933–1945* (New York: J. B. Lippincott Company, 1955) , p. 148.

3. Ibid., pp. 400–401.

4. *The Secret Diary of Harold L. Ickes* (New York: Simon & Schuster, 1954) , III, p. 208.

5. Theodore H. White, *The Making of the President, 1960* (New York: Atheneum House, 1961) , p. 278.

6. Ibid., p. 279.

7. Ickes, I, p. 573.

8. D. W. Brogan, *Politics in America* (New York: Harper & Row, Inc., 1954) , p. 271.

9. Hugh-Jones and Radice, p. 25.

10. Zetterburg, pp. 101–107.

11. Elmo Roper, *You and Your Leaders: Their Actions and Your Reactions, 1936–1956* (New York: William Morrow & Company, 1957) , p. 22.

12. "Conservatism," *Annals* of the American Academy of Political and Social Science, CCCXLIV (November, 1962), p. 14.

13. Brogan, p. 139.

14. See, for example, Jacques Barzun's perceptive volume on the role of science in modern culture, *Science: The Glorious Entertainment* (New York, 1964), especially the chapter on the behavioral sciences.

index